Antidepressants

Judy Monroe

—The Drug Library—

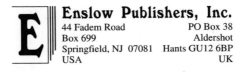

Enslow Publishers, Inc.

44 Fadem Road   PO Box 38
Box 699   Aldershot
Springfield, NJ 07081   Hants GU12 6BP
USA   UK

Library of Congress Cataloging-in-Publication Data

Monroe, Judy.
    Antidepressants / Judy Monroe.
        p. cm. — (The drug library)
    Includes bibliographical references (p.) and index.
    Summary: Examines the social and physical effects of antidepressants.
    ISBN 0-89490-848-0
    1. Antidepressants—Juvenile literature. [1. Antidepressants.]
  I. Title. II. Series.
  RM332.M66 1997
  616.85'27061—dc20
                                        96-23354
                                           CIP
                                         AC

Printed in the United States of America.

10 9 8 7 6 5 4 3 2 1

Photo Credits: Clay H. Bartl, pp. 30, 40, 43, 50, 57, 59, 77, 80, 95, 102, 106;
Depression Awareness, Recognition, and Treatment Program, Alcohol, Drug
Abuse, and Mental Health Administration, National Institute of Mental Health
Administration, U.S. Department of Health and Human Services, p. 14;
Depression Awareness, Recognition, and Treatment Program, Alcohol, Drug
Abuse, and Mental Health Administration, National Institute of Mental Health
Administration, U.S. Department of Health and Human Services, and National
Alliance for the Mentally Ill (NAMI), p. 66; Judy Monroe, p. 91; NAMI,
Arlington, VA, p. 18; NASA, p. 7; Suicide Awareness Voices of Education (SAVE),
Minneapolis, MN, p. 71.

Cover Photo: © Coco McCoy/Rainbow

Contents

1

Recovery from a Crippling Illness

In 1963 Colonel Edwin E. "Buzz" Aldrin, Jr., began training as a crew member for the history-making *Apollo 11* moon flight. The mission of the National Aeronautics Space Administration (NASA) was a first—to walk on the moon.

The *Apollo 11* astronauts underwent months of intense physical training and psychological testing. Healthy and fit, Aldrin easily passed all of his tests. On July 20, 1969, eighteen minutes after fellow astronaut Neil Armstrong left the *Apollo 11* lunar module, Aldrin became the second man to walk on the moon.

Crashing Down, Getting Back Up

The thrill and pride of achieving his dream did not last long for Aldrin, however. Back on Earth, Aldrin could not handle the emotional strain of being a celebrity. His stress level zoomed as he struggled with his busy schedule of parades, goodwill tours, and speaking engagements. He grew depressed and his confidence and self-esteem withered. Aldrin sometimes cried after speaking engagements. His fingers became numb and his neck ached. Finally, his depression overwhelmed him and he could no longer handle daily living. Aldrin recalled:

> I stopped. Stopped everything. I'd go to my office in the morning, determined to work a full day and then go home to more work. I'd sit down at my desk and stare out the window. A few hours would go by and I'd drive to the beach. . . . Then I'd go home for dinner, turn on the television, and get a bottle of Scotch. Or I'd not go home at all until everyone was in bed.[1]

Aldrin seemed to have everything: fame, money, and health. Yet he developed post-achievement depression, a type of depression brought on by success. Aldrin explained:

> I had gone to the moon. What to do next? What possible goal could I add now? There simply wasn't one, and without a goal I was like an inert ping-pong ball being batted about by the whims and motivations of others. I was suffering from what poets have described as the melancholy of all things done.[2]

To treat his depression, Aldrin received antidepressant medication and therapy. He eventually recovered.

6

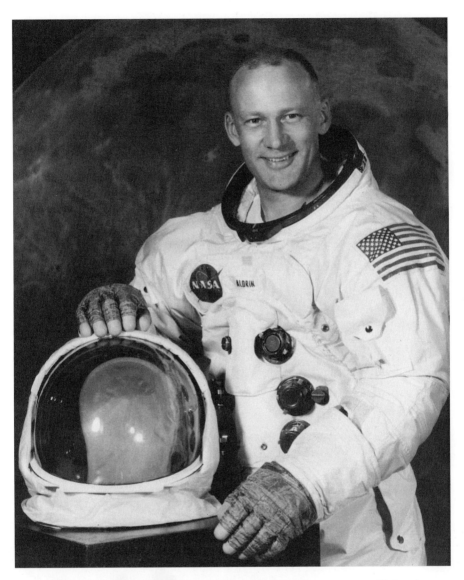

After achieving notable success, some people like astronaut Colonel Edwin E. "Buzz" Aldrin, Jr., develop depression. Aldrin eventually recovered from his illness with the help of antidepressant medications and psychotherapy.

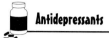

Antidepressants for Depression Treatment

Aldrin was lucky because he could get antidepressant medication to treat his depression. In the past, many people assumed that people with depression could not be helped or that a depressed person was weak.[3]

Research has since revealed that chemical changes in the brain, not personal weakness, can bring on depression. These chemical changes can be caused by some illnesses, certain medications, genetic factors, and environmental factors. Recently, researchers at the Washington University School of Medicine in St. Louis, Missouri, identified areas of the brain that function abnormally in depressed people. Dr. Wayne C. Drevets, assistant professor at the university, explained that these studies demonstrate that "major depression is a biological illness and not a case of people who are unable to keep their emotion in check because of some character weakness. Telling them to cheer up is not enough."[4]

This means that biology plays an important role in depression. So, antidepressant medications that affect the brain's functioning can help a depressed person feel better. The drugs decrease depressive symptoms and the risk of another depression surfacing. They can also improve a person's overall medical and emotional health.

The Blues

The word *depression* often has an unclear meaning in everyday use. Buzz Aldrin's depression, for example, is a medical disorder that can be treated, usually with antidepressant medication or a combination of antidepressant medications and psychotherapy. Feeling down or blue at a particular moment is not the same as depression. Kent (not his real name) described a recent day when he was feeling low.

> *I think I got up on the wrong side of the bed that morning. I just felt down. I'm a computer programmer and at work, I ran into a bug—that's a software problem—I couldn't fix. I forgot my lunch at home and overpaid for a lousy sandwich at the company cafeteria. The day crept by. By the time I got home from work, all I wanted to do was pull the blankets over my head and sleep until tomorrow. Which I did. What a difference the next day brought! I zipped into work, fixed the bug, and got twice as much done by lunch as I had all the day before. I felt like myself again.[5]*

Like Kent, most of us have periods of feeling blue for no reason. You might also feel down if bad weather cancels a long-awaited outdoor event or you got a low grade on a test that seemed easy. While struggling with negative thoughts, the hours drag by. It might be hard to get much done or be cheerful. These short periods of sadness are not true depression, however, and seldom require treatment.

Sometimes people suffer a deeper, longer period of sadness because of a shattering event. Losing a loved one, losing a job, or suffering serious injuries in an accident can send some people into deep sadness. Over time, people usually work out their feelings of grief and adjust to their loss.

Depths of Depression

In medical terms depression has a specific list of symptoms. There is no specific laboratory test for diagnosing depression.

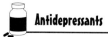

Instead, a health professional such as a doctor, psychiatrist, or clinical psychologist can help in making a diagnosis.

True depression is severe and requires treatment. It lasts longer than the blues, sometimes for months or years. Depression interferes with daily life, including family, friends, work, and school. It affects thoughts, feelings, physical health, and behaviors.

Common symptoms include negative and guilty feelings, weight gain or loss, and sleeping problems. In severe depression, people can have hallucinations (see or hear things that are not really there), withdraw from everyday activities, and lose touch with reality. Such depressions, said American psychiatrist Hugh Storrow, "probably cause more human suffering than any other single disease—mental or physical."[6] Depression symptoms differ from person to person. Three examples follow:

Elizabeth (not her real name) once balanced a job, marriage, and raising children. Now she cannot sleep at night and finds simple tasks nearly impossible to do. She once loved seeing plays and eating in restaurants, but she has lost interest in her former pleasures. Everyone is upset with Elizabeth— her husband, who is becoming impatient; her children, who feel abandoned and scared; and her boss, who warned her to shape up.[7]

Compared to Elizabeth, Nicole (not her real name) has not changed much in many years. She has always felt depressed and has not stuck with a job or finished college. Her husband left her with two small children, little money, and many angry words. Like Elizabeth, Nicole feels sad, guilty, and hopeless, but unlike Elizabeth, she sleeps and eats too much.[8]

Cathy (not her real name) clearly remembers what triggered her depression:

> *I had an extreme personal loss and I bottomed out. My loss was overwhelming and it triggered me to grieve over other past losses. I wasn't eating and I felt like my spirit was dead. I knew I needed some help and went to my doctor. After a month of antidepressant medication and therapy, I felt great!*[9]

Elizabeth, Nicole, and Cathy needed help to deal with their depression. Elizabeth, like many others, put off getting help because she hoped her sad feelings would disappear. When she started thinking about suicide as a way to escape her depression, her husband talked Elizabeth into seeing a doctor.

Focus on Depression

Depression is a mental illness. Its origins are usually biological, caused by a chemical imbalance in the brain. Anyone, at any age, including children and teens, can develop depression.

Because it affects the mind and personality, depressed people may feel ashamed or embarrassed. That is too bad, because depression is not a personality weakness or a moral lapse. People cannot "snap out of it." It is not the fault of the depressed person. As we better understand and treat this disease, the stigma of depression is subsiding. Annual national depression screenings are now held around the United States. Magazines and newspapers often run articles that explain depression and its symptoms and list places to go for help. People who have battled depression and have spoken out about their illness and recovery include: astronaut Colonel Edwin E. "Buzz" Aldrin, Jr.; CBS news correspondent Mike Wallace; actress Patty Duke; and Nobel Laureate in bacterial

11

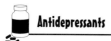

genetics Salvador Luria.[10] These people were lucky. Their symptoms were recognized, and they have all gone for treatment. Others are not as lucky.

According to the National Institute of Mental Health (NIMH) and the National Alliance for Research on Schizophrenia and Depression (NARSAD), 17.6 million Americans suffer from a depressive illness every year.[11] This ranks depression as the most common severe mental illness in the United States. Over thirty-five thousand Americans commit suicide each year, often before their depression is ever identified.[12] Suicide is the third leading cause of death among young people between the ages of fifteen to twenty-four and one of the leading causes of death among the elderly.[13]

Depression costs Americans $43.7 billion a year in treatment and lost work. Of that total, researchers calculate that depression generates $12.4 billion in medical bills a year.[14]

Antidepressant drugs have helped millions of people, but millions more still struggle with depression and have not sought help. Reluctance to get help sometimes springs from the false belief that "depression is a weak character or underlying laziness."[15] This fallacy is thousands of years old.

Researchers estimate that only one-third of depressed people seek treatment. Yet most depressed people—80 to 90 percent—can be helped by antidepressants and/or therapy.[16] Once treated, many will never have another period of depression, especially if antidepressant treatment begins early.

Recovery with Antidepressants

Many organizations provide education programs about depression, offer treatment, or provide referrals. Most depressed people can get control of their illness and enjoy a full life. One way to do this is through the use of antidepressant medications.

Antidepressants are prescription medications that prevent or relieve depression. Doctors prescribe them to treat depressed people of all ages. These drugs help the brain of people who are depressed to produce important, but missing, neurochemicals, or to keep these neurochemicals from breaking down too soon. The United States Food and Drug Administration (FDA) regulates all antidepressant medications.

Doctors can now prescribe from over twenty different antidepressants. Because of similar chemical makeup, antidepressants fall into one of three main classes or groups: cyclic antidepressants, monamine oxidase inhibitors (MAOIs), and selective serotonin reuptake inhibitors (SSRIs). A few other chemically different antidepressants that do not fit these groups are also available. There is a lot of overlap in their actions and uses, but these three different classes work differently, have different side effects, and may be favored by doctors and those taking a medication for varying reasons.

Antidepressant medications have not been around for very long. The first one was introduced in the mid-1950s. Considering the short time they have been available, antidepressant medications have helped to bring about great changes in the treatment of depression. People who, years ago, might have spent time in mental hospitals because of their depression can now receive antidepressant medication to take each day, while they lead their regular lives.

One important benefit from antidepressant medications is a greater understanding of the causes of depression. Scientists have learned a great deal more about the workings of the brain due to

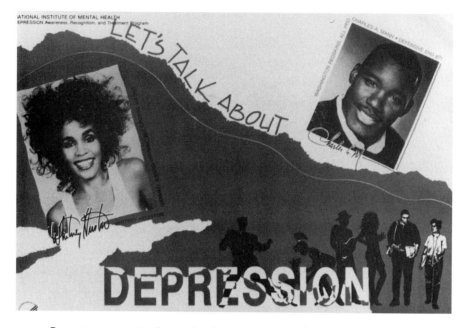

Recent progress in the study of depression has focused on treatment, particularly with antidepressant medications.

their research into how antidepressants relieve depression. Antidepressant medications also may make other kinds of treatment more useful. Someone who is too depressed to talk, for example, cannot get much benefit from psychotherapy or counseling. For many, the right antidepressant improves the symptoms of depression so that they can better tackle their problems and enjoy life again.

Questions for Discussion

1. How would you feel if you found out your best friend was taking an antidepressant to treat depression?

2. What do you do for yourself when you feel down or blue?

3. Why do you think people have such mixed feelings about how to deal with depression?

2

History of Antidepressants

According to Hippocrates, the Greek "Father of Medicine" (460 B.C. to 375 B.C.), depression was a disease of the mind. During depression, he said, an imbalance of bodily fluids called humors occurred, and extra black bile was produced. Herbs and minerals were used to counteract the extra bile and to treat the depression.

Although his treatments seldom helped, Hippocrates was on the right track. Today we know that a chemical imbalance in the brain is often the cause of depression. However, chemistry had not been invented in Hippocrates's time. Thousands of years went by before a breakthrough in treating depression was

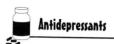
Abraham Lincoln *Virginia Woolf* **Lionel Aldridge** *Eugene O'Neill* **Beethoven**
Gaetano Donizetti *Robert Schumann* LEO TOLSTOY *Vaslov Nijinsky*
John Keats Tennessee Williams **Vincent Van Gogh** Isaac Newton **Ernest Hemingway**
Sylvia Plath Michelangelo WINSTON CHURCHILL *Vivien Leigh*
Emperor Norton I Jimmy Piersall Patty Duke **Charles Dickens**

PEOPLE WITH MENTAL ILLNESSES
ENRICH OUR LIVES.

These people have experienced one of the major mental illnesses of Schizophrenia, Manic-Depression and/or Major Depression.

To understand more, call 1-800-950-NAMI.

@NAMI

NATIONAL ALLIANCE FOR THE MENTALLY ILL

Because of their severe depression and lack of treatment, famous writers such as Ernest Hemingway, Sylvia Plath, and Virginia Woolf committed suicide.

made—the first antidepressants were discovered. The first antidepressants were actually designed to treat other illnesses. Doctors stumbled upon their positive effects on depression by accident in the early 1950s.

The First Tricyclic Antidepressant

In 1952 the introduction of a drug used to treat schizophrenia launched the tricyclic antidepressants (TCAs). Schizophrenia is a mental illness in which a person loses awareness of reality and the ability to relate closely with others. It is often associated with problems of behavior and the lack of ability to reason. Researchers had hoped that this drug would also treat depression, but tests for this were unsuccessful.[1] CIBA Geigy, the Swiss company that owned the drug, changed it slightly and called it G22355.

CIBA Geigy asked Dr. Roland Kuhn, a Swiss psychiatrist, to test the effectiveness of this new drug in treating depression. Since Kuhn was seeking a workable antidepressant medication, he began experimenting with G22355 in 1956. First he gave it to three people with severe depression. When all three improved within a month, Kuhn continued testing with good results.

In 1957 Kuhn presented his results with G22355 at the Second International Congress of Psychiatry in Zurich, Switzerland. Less than twelve people attended the Congress. Kuhn was not discouraged by this poor turnout or by the chilly reception toward his findings. He recalled, "Our paper was received with a great deal of skepticism. This was not surprising in view of the almost completely negative history of the drug treatment of depression up to that time."[2] Word of Kuhn's success with the new drug quickly spread, and other European psychiatrists began prescribing it for depression. In 1958 the drug was introduced into the United States and soon was widely used to treat people with severe depression.

Tricyclics and Other Cyclics

Other European and American drug companies rushed to develop their own cyclic antidepressants. Elavil™ (amitriptyline) was released next. Elavil is a tricyclic antidepressant. Since then, six other tricyclic medications have been approved in the United States to treat depression. Scientists have also developed four slightly different cyclics. All twelve drugs are members of the cyclic class or group of antidepressants.

Origins of MAOIs

About the same time the first tricyclic antidepressant was born, the first MAOIs were also discovered. MAOIs trace their roots to an antibiotic drug used to treat tuberculosis. Tuberculosis is an infectious disease that affects mainly the lungs. Introduced in 1951, the drug gave many people with tuberculosis added benefits: It heightened their mood and increased their sense of well-being. Doctors recorded this information in their published medical papers.

Five years passed before someone thought to use this drug as an antidepressant. That person was Dr. Nathan Kline, an American researcher who was searching for a drug to lift depression. This yet unknown drug, he said at a 1956 American Psychoanalytic Association presentation, would, "reduce the sleep requirements and delay the onset of fatigue. It would increase appetite and sexual desire and increase behavioral drive in general. Motor and intellectual activity would be speeded up. It would heighten responsiveness to stimuli [and] would result in a sense of joyousness and optimism."[3]

One week after his presentation, Kline was in New Jersey giving a lecture. Afterward a researcher told him of his experiments with rats and two drugs. One drug energized the rats. Kline researched the medical literature and found that many doctors had noticed this drug's energizing effects on people with tuberculosis.

Kline began testing the researcher's drug. His first study was with nine depressed people. One did not respond, another showed little improvement, but the other seven soon showed great improvement. He continued testing with impressive results. As news of Kline's experiments spread, other researchers confirmed the antidepressant effects of this drug. The Food and Drug Administration soon approved the medication to treat depression. Use of the drug was later abandoned because it can cause jaundice, a condition of not enough bile in the body, which turns skin, tissues, and body fluids yellow. Its discovery, however, led to the discovery of related antidepressants, called MAOIs, to combat depression. Today three MAOIs are prescribed in the United States.

Building a New Type of Antidepressant

Although the older cyclic and MAOI antidepressants worked well, they often caused side effects and took weeks or months before becoming effective. Researchers wanted to develop new antidepressants that would work faster and have fewer side effects.[4] The search for a new type of antidepressant was launched in 1971 by three researchers at Eli Lilly and Company: Bryan B. Molloy, Ray Fuller, and Dave Wong. These three men and hundreds of other researchers took more than fifteen years to develop and test their new drug. Molloy, an organic chemist, directed the project.

Molloy and his research team decided to try a different route to come up with a new antidepressant. In the past, many new drugs for depression were discovered when doctors prescribed them for one illness, but noticed that the drugs also helped those who had a second illness, depression. The researchers at Lilly instead targeted a specific chemical imbalance in the brain that seemed to cause depression. They also decided that their new drug would not have many of the less desirable side effects of the older antidepressants. Molloy recalled that in 1971, at the

21

beginning of the project, "When we started off on this journey, it's true that we didn't know exactly where we were going, but it got clearer as the experiment went along."[5]

They first examined the various antihistamines that Lilly had stored in its vaults for research purposes. Antihistamines are drugs that relieve the symptoms of allergies or colds by blocking the production or action of histamines. Histamines cause runny, itchy eyes and a runny nose. They started with antihistamines because the older antidepressants chemically resemble antihistamines. The researchers changed the antihistamines, then tested and retested them. Less than two years later, they created a substance that met their requirements. The researchers named the new medication Prozac™ and created a new class of antidepressants called Selective Serotonin Reuptake Inhibitors (SSRIs).

More Testing

Before Lilly could sell Prozac, the medication went through years of testing to meet approval by the FDA. The FDA is a government agency that approves all medications used in the United States. Years of early testing on animals and healthy human volunteers showed good results. In the late 1970s, new studies with Prozac were launched on thousands of depressed people. During these studies, researchers found that this drug might also help those with other mental disorders. Much larger groups of people with depression were tested next.

More than eleven years of testing had gone by. On September 6, 1983, Lilly submitted a new-drug request to the FDA. The FDA examined all the paperwork from the eleven years of testing and recommended that Prozac be approved to treat depression. Four more years went by. Finally, on December 29, 1987, the FDA approved Prozac for use in the United States.

Used Worldwide

During the FDA's examination time, Prozac was already widely used in Belgium and South Africa. By the late 1980s, the medication was allowed in most countries around the world. By 1990, Prozac ranked as the world's most widely prescribed antidepressant.[6] Sales zoomed up as television talk shows and national magazines declared it a wonder drug. Sales dropped somewhat in 1991, however, when critics lashed out against the drug. They claimed that the drug caused some people to commit suicide.

Eli Lilly and Company defended its medication. The FDA reexamined information on Prozac and in October 1991, declared it a safe and useful drug to treat depression. Since then, Prozac has again sold well. In fact, the drug ranks fifth in sales among all prescription drugs in the United States.[7] So far, over twelve million people around the world have taken Prozac.[8]

Growing Numbers of Antidepressants

Two other antidepressants, chemical cousins to Prozac, soon followed. In December 1990, Paxil™, made by SmithKline Beecham Pharmaceuticals received FDA approval for treating depression. Some European countries and Canada had already approved Paxil. In December 1991, the FDA approved Zoloft™, which was already used in Great Britain for treating depression.

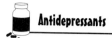

Pfizer, Inc. manufactures Zoloft. Today Zoloft ranks second to Prozac in sales, while Paxil ranks third.

The appearance of Effexor™ in 1993 by Wyeth-Ayerst Laboratories Company launched another new type of antidepressant. It is chemically different from any of the other antidepressants. Effexor falls into the class of antidepressants called Serotonin Nonselective Reuptake Inhibitors (SNRIs). It works much like the other antidepressants but seems to have fewer side effects than older antidepressants.

Questions for Discussion

1. Since the late 1800s, nervous breakdown has been a phrase used to mean an extremely serious depression. How do you think this phrase came into use?

2. Why do you think so many drug companies develop their own versions of antidepressants?

3. More women than men tend to suffer from depression. Why do you think this is true?

3

Physical Effects of Antidepressants

Just as aspirin can reduce a fever without clearing up the infection that causes it, antidepressants act by controlling the symptoms of depression, without curing the actual causes of the depression. Like most drugs used as medication, antidepressants correct or make up for some malfunction in the body. They do not cure a person who is depressed. Instead, they lessen the burden by lifting the dark, heavy moods of depression. They also relieve the physical symptoms, such as sleep problems or poor appetite. Antidepressants help people get on with life.

Controversy over Antidepressants

Unfortunately, some people still attach a stigma to the use of antidepressants as a treatment for depression. A 1993 Gallup poll found that 25 percent of Americans would say no to taking an antidepressant if they were depressed.[1]

Perhaps some of this negativity comes from a misunderstanding of what antidepressants actually do. Because these drugs cause changes in the brain, some people think they would develop a different personality if they took an antidepressant.[2]

Simon (not his real name), for example, felt uneasy when his doctor recommended an antidepressant. "I was flooded with emotions: shock, outrage, and underneath it all, shame . . . I must be really sick (and therefore bad) if he thinks I need medication."[3] Simon felt that he had failed since he could not recover on his own from his depression. He recalled, "What would people say or think when I told them I took antidepressants?"[4]

Gabrielle (not her real name) too, had to change her attitude toward antidepressants. She had struggled with depression for over a decade. Finally, she asked for help. When her doctor suggested an antidepressant, Gabrielle replied, "I believe this medication can help me, but I'm afraid it will change me."[5] Her doctor's reply was reassuring. "It will change you. You'll be you again."[6]

Overall, people's attitudes about the use of antidepressants are changing. More people are willing to accept the help that antidepressants can give. Dr. Daniel X. Freedman at the University of California at Los Angeles confirmed this attitude shift. "You see fewer patients who pit themselves against the medicine, as if their integrity or ability to exercise willpower were at issue."[7]

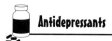

Benefits and Drawbacks of Antidepressant Medications

Antidepressant medications offer three main benefits in treating depression:

1. They are easy for a doctor to prescribe.

2. They have been proven to help those with mild, moderate, and severe depression.

3. People do not need a lot of time to take the medications.

These medications also have at least eight drawbacks. These include:

1. The need for repeated doctor visits to monitor the person's response and perhaps adjust the dose.

2. Side effects can occur.

3. Although less frequent, more severe medical reactions such as an allergic reaction of hives or an itchy rash can occur.

4. There is the potential for their use in suicide attempts by the person who is depressed.

5. Failure of many people—10 to 30 percent—to complete the antidepressant medication treatment.

6. Antidepressants do not help every person with depression.

7. The person must stick to the medication schedule.

8. Some people will need to continue taking antidepressant medication for years or a lifetime.

For many depressed people the benefits of treatment with antidepressant medications far outweigh the risks or inconveniences.

What Antidepressants Do

People taking antidepressants do not get high. Most people are not aware of being on a medication, except that their depressive symptoms become less intense and they function better.[8] The benefits of antidepressants can take several weeks or more to become apparent. Sometimes the changes are not obvious.[9] People who take antidepressants do not escape, ignore, or become numb to their problems.

One of the first improvements people notice when taking antidepressants is improved sleep. They get more restful sleep, often with fewer nightmares. The antidepressant also increases energy and ability to concentrate and perks up decreased appetites. People become more alert and less tired. Emotional improvements will also be noticeable. People find that their negative thinking and sadness begin to lift. Chuck (not his real name) explains:

> I didn't know that I was depressed . . . But I had a terrible feeling of doom that followed me all the time. When I went to see a psychiatrist, he had me take some tests. My depression scores were so high they nearly went off the charts! My psychiatrist prescribed amitriptyline [Elavil]. I didn't feel any different when I started taking this antidepressant. But within weeks, that feeling of doom lifted. And I could now fall asleep quickly and slept soundly the whole night.[10]

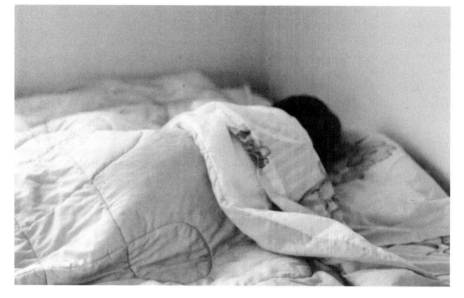

Sleeping too much is a typical symptom of major depression. Once people start taking antidepressant medication, they can resume their normal sleeping patterns.

Antidepressants do not change people dramatically or make them forget their problems. Dr. Patricia Owen of the Hazelden Foundation explained that many people who take antidepressants say the drugs do not change their lives directly but make them feel normal again. They still feel disappointments and good things. These medications, she said, "provide a stable foundation so [people] can make changes."[11]

While on antidepressants, Tanya (not her real name) did not change into a different person, but she found that she could better cope with her problems. Tanya had been depressed for a long time before she tried an antidepressant. She found that the drug made a difference.

*I seemed to be more tolerant of others and less judgmental
of myself, and I felt I was making pretty good decisions. . . .
I don't mean to say that it was a huge difference, that everything was rosy, but it was different. I could handle things
better.*[12]

Tanya summed up her experience on antidepressants:

*Meds won't cure you by themselves. You are still responsible
for your actions or lack of actions. And it's difficult to do the
things you need to do for yourself . . . Maybe meds can help,
but just like anything else, it only works when you work it.*[13]

Antidepressants are not Addicting

Experts report that antidepressants are not addictive. They are
not stimulants or uppers, they do not make someone happy.
Antidepressants only work for people who are depressed, by
improving their mood. An addiction occurs when someone
develops a psychological or physical dependence on a drug.
Most addicts develop tolerance to a drug. They need higher and
higher doses to get the same effect. People on antidepressants do
not require higher doses, and they do not form a dependence on
the medication. Also, the mood-improving effects of antidepressants develop slowly over weeks or months, unlike addictive
drugs that work quickly, often within minutes or hours.

Although LaVon's (not her real name) doctor recommended
an antidepressant, she kept hesitating. LaVon realized that she
felt antidepressants were addicting, because LaVon's mother said
she loved her antidepressant. LaVon agreed to try an antidepressant
when her doctor, "pointed out that people didn't get high on

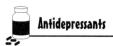

antidepressants; it was just a way to overcome a chemical imbalance in your brain."[14]

Which One to Take?

Antidepressants are most widely used for serious depression and are only sometimes prescribed for milder depression. Doctors decide which antidepressant to prescribe for someone. They base their selection on how severe the depression is, the type of depression, a person's age and overall health, possible side effects of the antidepressant, and the chance of interactions with other drugs the person may be taking.

Another factor that can help in the selection of an antidepressant is how other family members have responded to particular antidepressants. Research has shown that responses to antidepressants may run in families. So, if a person has a parent, brother, or sister who responded well to one antidepressant, this medication or a similar one may be a good first try.

Like any medication, antidepressants do not produce the same effects in everyone. Some people respond better to one medication than another. Some may need larger dosages than others. Some experience annoying, unwanted side effects, while others do not. Various factors can influence the effects of an antidepressant, including age, gender, body size, body chemistry, and diet. Since there is no certain way to determine which medication will be the best, the doctor may have to prescribe first one, than another, until the one that works is found.

To increase the odds that an antidepressant will do its job, people must work with their doctor. They need to tell the doctor about their past medical history and any other medications they are taking (including non-prescription medications). After taking the drug for awhile, they need to report any side effects. Psychotherapy may also help the person to talk over their personal issues.

Angie's (not her real name) first antidepressant gave her mixed results. After seeing a doctor about her depression, Angie took Tofranil™, a cyclic antidepressant. Although it helped lessen her depression, she could not deal with its side effects. She then tried Prozac. This drug also worked to make her symptom-free of depression, but with no side effects.

Over twenty antidepressants are currently available in the United States. They differ in their side effects and, to some extent, in how successfully they control the symptoms of depression.

To treat depression, doctors generally prescribe the cyclic antidepressants and the SSRIs. The MAOIs often help those with depression whose atypical symptoms include oversleeping, anxiety, panic attacks, and phobias.

Is There a Best One?

Doctors rate the various antidepressants at about the same levels of effectiveness when they are used to treat depression. After analyzing over four hundred studies of antidepressants, the Depression Guideline Panel said, "no one antidepressant is clearly more effective than another."[15] The United States Department of Health and Human Services assembled the Depression Guideline Panel in the early 1990s. This panel determines suggested treatment guidelines and is made up of health experts.

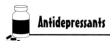

No doctor can predict which antidepressant will work best for someone. Scientists are trying to develop laboratory tests to determine the best medication for each person, but they have not yet had any success. Doctors generally take a trial and error approach. "Antidepressant treatment clearly is not a question of one pill for everything and everyone," said Colette Dowling, a speaker on mental health.[16] Doctors usually prescribe an antidepressant that they have had success with and think will work well. According to the American Pharmaceutical Association, between 20 and 30 percent of people fail to respond to the first antidepressant they take.[17] Other experts say that figure is higher, at 40 to 50 percent.[18]

Treatment Plans

When someone begins taking an antidepressant, generally they will not see improvement right away. With most antidepressants, it usually takes from several weeks to a month or more before noticeable changes occur.[19] Researchers do not know why it takes this length of time before antidepressants begin to work. Some symptoms lessen early in treatment, while others diminish later. For example, a person's energy level or sleeping or eating patterns may improve before his or her depressed mood lifts. If there is little or no change in symptoms after five or six weeks, the doctor may increase the dosage or amount of antidepressant taken or prescribe a different antidepressant.

The standard dosage for each antidepressant varies. Dosage depends on the type of antidepressant and the person's body chemistry, age, and weight. Doctors generally start with low dosages. This allows the body to gradually adjust to the drug.

The dosage is slowly raised over time until the desired effect is reached. The doctor may also monitor the level of the drug in the person's blood. Such monitoring enables the doctor to determine if the person is taking too much of the medication. Monitoring also helps reduce the chance of side effects.

In younger people, effects of an antidepressant can show up within several weeks. In older people, it can take longer for an antidepressant to reduce depression.[20] Researchers still have not discovered the reason for the discrepancy in reactions between age groups.

Sometimes people decide their antidepressant is not working well, but actually they have not given it enough time. Usually it takes two months before one can assess if an antidepressant works. Since many people start with low dosages and gradually increase over time, this two-month period starts from the time of the last dose increase.

To get the best results, people need to take their medication as prescribed. Writing down the doctor's instructions helps. Here are six things that someone taking an antidepressant needs to ask the doctor or pharmacist:

- *What should be done if I miss a scheduled dose, or even a day of medication?*
- *What other medications can interact with the antidepressant to cause serious problems?*
- *What side effects can occur and how should they be managed if they appear?*
- *What side effects are serious enough to merit a call to the doctor?*
- *What are the signs that the antidepressant is beginning to work?*

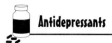

• *How long will it take before I experience the full
benefit of the drug?*

Length of Treatment

Once an antidepressant is controlling the depression, determining
how long to remain on the medication is different for each individual. If antidepressants are stopped too soon, the person can
relapse or have another bout of depression. The length of time
needed for antidepressant treatment varies from person to person. Some researchers find that continuing medication even after
depression has lifted can prevent future episodes from occurring.

The National Institute of Mental Health Depression
Collaborative Research Program found that four months of treatment with antidepressants is not enough for most depressed
people to fully recover and remain symptom-free. Generally,
doctors treat most people for at least six to twelve months to
prevent a relapse.[21] Some people take an antidepressant for more
than a year. Research has shown that the first eight weeks after
the symptoms of depression are gone is the riskiest time for
another depressive episode to occur.[22]

Among those who take an antidepressant for a year or less,
50 percent have just that one episode of depression and never
have another one.[23] They may also remain symptom-free for
years before going through another episode of depression. The
period of time during which a person is depressed is called an
episode of depression. Episodes usually have a definite beginning
and an end.

Beth (not her real name) needed an antidepressant for a short
time. Everything was going well for her, but then she started

having problems at work. She developed sleeping problems, had no appetite, and withdrew from coworkers and friends. Beth went to a psychiatrist who prescribed the antidepressant Paxil. Although skeptical, she tried the drug and found that it brought back her self-confidence and made her more capable. She stopped taking the drug after eight months and has not needed an antidepressant since then.[24]

Antidepressants for Life

Other people find that their depression becomes more frequent and severe over time. For these people, continuing or maintenance treatment with antidepressants can reduce or eliminate the episodes of depression. According to Dr. Mark S. Gold at the University of Florida College of Medicine, the odds are very good that antidepressants can keep a person symptom-free for life.[25]

Fred (not his real name) is an example. After Fred lost his longtime job, he started teaching and consulting. But when Fred and his wife took a trip to Europe, he disappeared one morning. He was found three days later, sitting in a small village, crying and unable to speak. His wife got him back to the United States and into a hospital. After Fred was diagnosed with both depression and shock from losing his longtime job, he began taking an antidepressant. His life eventually returned to normal.[26]

Fred later went off the antidepressant and within a year became extremely depressed again. He went to see Dr. Gold who told Fred that by taking antidepressants for the rest of his life, he would remain symptom-free. But Fred did not want to take antidepressant medication every day.[27]

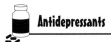

Because Fred had two episodes of depression in less than one year, he would need to take antidepressants for life. Dr. Gold explained to Fred that he had a recurring disease that would be with him all of his life. "It wasn't a question of 'When will I be cured?' or 'When can I stop taking antidepressants?' but rather, 'Why risk the chance of becoming depressed again?'"[28] Fred has stayed on antidepressants and once again leads a symptom-free life.

Dr. Lawrence Cohen at the Oklahoma Health Sciences Center added that those who use antidepressants on a continuing basis need to understand that the medication is not temporary. Because they will never be cured, they will not go off of the antidepressant someday. "While that would be the ideal, there is nothing wrong with being on a medication the rest of one's life, if it will assure a better quality of life and it truly is needed," he said.[29]

Side Effects

Side effects are unintended but fairly common effects produced by medications. Each antidepressant produces various side effects in people. No two people will experience exactly the same side effects in exactly the same way, even if they are taking the same medication, at the same dosage. Every prescription medication, including antidepressants, can cause unwanted reactions. Not all antidepressants produce all side effects, and not everybody gets them. People who are taking antidepressants need to discuss all symptoms and side effects with a doctor. If side effects are especially troublesome, the doctor can change the dosage or medication.

Arnette (not her real name) tried four antidepressants, including SSRIs, over two years. She gained ten pounds with each antidepressant, although SSRIs sometimes cause people to lose weight. When she complained to her doctor, he replied that "taking the medication was a double-edged sword."[30] He meant that there are both good and bad aspects to it. Unsatisfied, Arnette responded, "So what is one suppose to do? Be happy and fat . . . or depressed and skinny? Not much choice."[31]

She decided to stop taking the antidepressants. She soon lost the forty extra pounds, but the symptoms of her severe depression returned. This time, her doctor tried a different antidepressant, and Arnette exercised and ate healthy, low-fat foods. She decided to live with any weight gain caused by the antidepressant.

Some side effects can be similar to the original symptoms of depression, such as fatigue and constipation. One common side effect of many of the antidepressants is "feeling foggy, dizzy, or overly medicated."[32] Taking the antidepressant only at bedtime can help to relieve this.

Although side effects can be unpleasant, most are not life-threatening. Antidepressants differ in both the number of people in whom they produce side effects, and in their range of side effects. Tricyclic antidepressants, for example, cause many people to develop a dry mouth and eyes. Some side effects are more common at the start of treatment and often disappear after two or three weeks. If side effects are particularly troublesome, the doctor may switch antidepressant medications.

Every couple of years, Jane Doe (not her real name) would get extremely depressed. Between episodes, she had low-level, chronic depression. She first tried Tofranil™, a tricyclic antidepressant. But she had many side effects, including blurry vision and constipation. Then she read about Prozac and asked her doctor to prescribe it for her. This antidepressant has worked well for Jane. She said, "I have never been tempted to go off Prozac . . . For me, it adjusts my brain chemistry and I am sure that I am going to be on it for the rest of my life."[33]

Combining Antidepressants

Sometimes depressed people take more than one type of antidepressant at a time. For those whose depression is not responding to any one antidepressant, a doctor may suggest a combination therapy of a cyclic antidepressant and an MAOI. A thyroid supplemement also increases the effectiveness of some cyclic

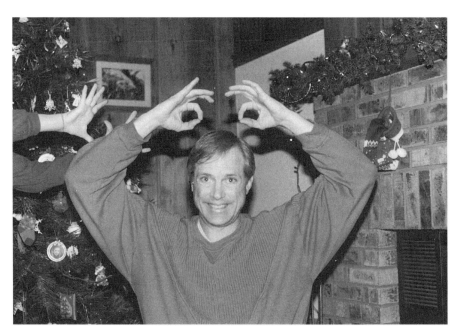

People with chronic mild depression can be helped to get on with their lives with antidepressants.

antidepressants. Scientists do not yet know why the thyroid impacts on how well an antidepressant works. One psychiatrist explained that, "A depressed person whose thyroid gland is the slightest bit underactive will respond poorly to antidepressants."[34] So, sometimes doctors will add a small dose of thyroid medication along with the antidepressant.

Not all antidepressants can be safely combined. Sometimes the different antidepressants will interact negatively and can cause serious problems. For example, some cyclic antidepressants can interact with MAOIs and produce fever, seizures, and even death. Combining an SSRI and an MAOI can bring on chills, fever, skin rash, restlessness, seizures, and fatigue—or even worse, the person could die after falling into a coma. Doctors are trained to know which antidepressants can be safely combined.

Drug Interactions

Because of possible interactions between various antidepressants, sometimes people must wait a while before switching from one antidepressant to another. This is called a washout period. The person stops taking one antidepressant, waits a few weeks, then can begin taking a different antidepressant.

Doctors often recommend a two-week washout period when switching from one type of antidepressant to another. A longer washout period of five to six weeks is needed for particular switches, such as when going from Prozac to an MAOI. It takes that long for all of the Prozac to leave the body.[35]

Sometimes antidepressants interact with other unrelated medications that someone is taking. This can cause the antidepressants to work poorly or not at all. Quite a few drugs can

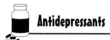

interact with antidepressants. Examples include drugs to treat high blood pressure, arthritis, lung problems, migraines, and seizures. Women who take drugs to treat breast cancer often cannot use antidepressants because the drugs tend to interact negatively.[36]

How Antidepressants Work

Researchers still do not know exactly how antidepressants work. The current theory is that antidepressants increase the amount of certain chemicals called neurotransmitters in the brain. Nerve cells in the brain create the neurotransmitters. Neurotransmitters send electrical signals or messages from nerve cell to nerve cell. When they finish carrying out their tasks, the neurotransmitters are broken down by enzymes, and reabsorbed by the nerve cells that originally released them. If reabsorbed or broken down too fast, not enough of these neurotransmitters remain in the brain. This low level of neurotransmitters appears to cause depression by affecting behavior, feelings, and thoughts.

Scientists have targeted their research to two specific transmitters: serotonin and norepinephrine. If the levels of these neurotransmitters in the brain drop too low, mood drops, along with the need for sleep and food. Activity and speech also slow down and self-esteem falls.[37]

Antidepressants strengthen the action of serotonin and norepinephrine. Each of the three antidepressant categories does this differently. The cyclics work by blocking the reabsorption of serotonin and norepinephrine by the nerve cells that released them. This raises the level of serotonin and norepinephrine in the brain and improves the electrical signals between the nerve cells. Normal mood is then restored.

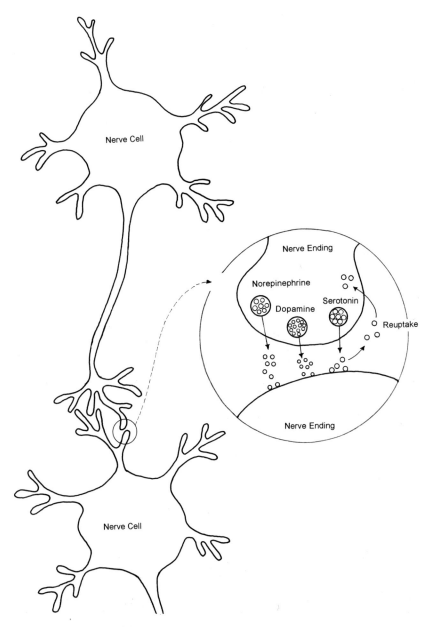

Nerve cells produce neurotransmitters to relay information on to the next nerve cells. Once the neurotransmitters have done their job, they are reabsorbed by the originating nerve cell. Antidepressants slow down the reuptake or reabsorption process.

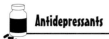

MAOIs differ in their actions. They hold back the enzymes that break down serotonin and norpinephrine. So, MAOIs allow more of these two chemicals to remain in the brain, which restores normal mood.

The newer antidepressants, the SSRIs, work much like the cyclics. They, too, block reabsorption, but only of one neurotransmitter, serotonin. This keeps serotonin circulating longer and depression is lifted. Dr. James Halikas at the University of Minnesota explained that the cyclics deliver a "shotgun" approach compared to the SSRIs, which are like "using a bullet."[38]

Safety

When taken as directed, antidepressants are safe. Beyond annoying side effects, they do not cause most people serious problems. Since the tricyclic antidepressants and MAOIs have a track record of over thirty years, doctors have compiled the most safety information about these drugs. The long-term safety of SSRIs and SNRIs is still relatively unknown because they have only been available since the 1980s.

Recently, researchers found evidence that low to mid-level doses of Prozac and Elavil, two of the most popular antidepressants, may cause tumors to grow more quickly. A group of Canadian scientists reported that when rodents were given Prozac and Elavil, their breast cancer and other tumors increased in weight and size. Until more research is done on this issue, researcher Dr. Jimmie Holland at the Memorial Sloan-Kettering Cancer Center in New York City recommends that people with depression and tumors or cancer should take their antidepressants. "Depression is a problem that needs aggressive treatment. Many breast cancer patients who should be recognized as depressed remain untreated"[39]

Generic Antidepressants

Some of the older antidepressants are also available as generic drugs. Generic drugs are similar to the brand-name medications, but with small differences. Are they as good as the brand-name antidepressants? The answer is sometimes. Generic drugs generally cost a lot less than the brand-name antidepressants. But they do vary slightly from the original brand-name drug. Under the FDA's standards, they can contain more or less of the active ingredients and of the additives or inert (nonactive) ingredients.

A drug company assigns its antidepressant both a generic name—a name related to its chemical makeup—and a trade or brand name. If the antidepressant is called by its trade name, the symbol ™ appears after the name, which stands for trademark.

Although the active ingredient (the actual trade-name antidepressant) remains the same in a brand name and its generic drug, the FDA allows many variables. Added ingredients such as binders, fillers, color, and flavoring can differ, along with the manufacturing process. These variables can affect how much of the drug enters the bloodstream and how quickly it moves into the brain.

Sometimes people who switch from a trade name antidepressant to a generic can get too little or too much of the active ingredient. Their depression may then return due to underdosing. They could also become extremely ill from overdosing. In general, generic antidepressants work well, because all medications undergo monitoring by the FDA. However, users should contact

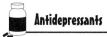

their doctor if they are uncertain. If someone has taken the same antidepressant for a while with good results, and suddenly has problems after a prescription is renewed, perhaps a generic antidepressant was switched for the trade-name antidepressant, or vice versa.

If someone finds that their depression is controlled by a particular generic prescription, they should get the manufacturer's name from the pharmacist. Then they can always request the same manufacturer's drug each time the prescription is filled.

Future Answers

According to the National Alliance for Research on Schizophrenia and Depression (NARSAD), for those treated with antidepressants, 20 to 30 percent will get no relief from their depression. NARSAD also stated that among those who respond well to antidepressant treatment, future episodes of depression "are not uncommon."[40]

More research is needed into these issues. The National Institute of Mental Health, other federal organizations, and private research groups such as NARSAD are running studies on antidepressants. These studies will help researchers better understand how and why antidepressants work and how to make these drugs work even better. They also will better learn how to control or eliminate unwanted side effects.

Questions for Discussion

1. Examine your own feelings and beliefs about mental illness. Do you have any stereotypes or prejudices?

2. Sometimes we feel like nothing is going right. Whom do you talk to when you feel this way? Are there other people you can turn to?

3. Why do you think that some people need to take antidepressants for months, but others need to continue taking antidepressants for life?

4

Young People and Antidepressants

Treatment for young people who are depressed sometimes includes antidepressant medications. No one knows how many young people are receiving antidepressant medications today. We do know, however, how many young people suffer from depression that probably requires treatment. The National Alliance for the Mentally Ill estimates that about 2 percent of children and 5 percent of teens in the United States suffer from depression.[1]

Medical doctor Lawrence L. Kerns, a specialist in childhood depression, thinks those numbers are low. "As many as 6 million children and adolescents in the United States—about 10 percent—are depressed. Not just a little blue or sad once in a while, or bored, or lonely, or worried, but suffering from a serious and potentially fatal illness: depression," according to Kerns.[2]

Youth and Antidepressants

Until the early 1980s, most health professionals did not believe that young people could suffer from depression.[3] As a result, few teens received antidepressants for treatment of depression. During the 1980s, researchers began to unravel the biochemistry of depression. They started to ask if young people, as well as adults, could have this illness. Their studies have shown that children and teens do get depressed and also have other mood disorders, such as obsessive-compulsive disorder (OCD).

One problem in diagnosing depression in young people is that the signs of depression are often not recognized. Depressed teens may not look sad or depressed but instead may talk about blunted feelings. Many express their feelings by taking action such as skipping school, running away from home, or turning to violence. Some teens turn to alcohol or drugs to deal with the sadness from their depression. Others slip into depression because of alcohol and drug abuse. Self-medicating with alcohol or other drugs may make a teen feel better for the moment but soon brings additional problems.

Do teens know if they are depressed? "That varies," said Dr. Ralph Rovner, a licensed clinical psychologist who works with depressed young people. He explains:

> *Teens are concerned about being normal. They want to establish their own identity and to view themselves as fitting in with others. Teens may deny their depression or just not be aware of it. Others might say that they're unhappy. Sometimes a child or teen will say to a parent, counselor, or teacher, "I hate myself and I'd rather be dead," or "I want to be dead."*[4]

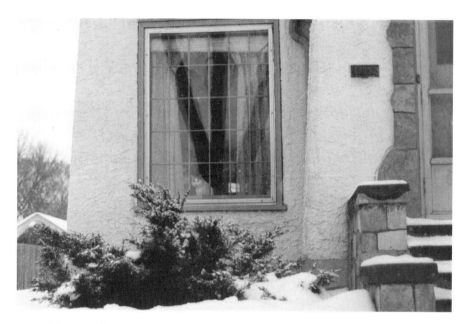

Untreated depression in teens can result in alcohol and drug abuse, risky sexual behavior, running away from home, or even suicide.

Changes in habits and personality that last more than two weeks are important clues in teen depression. Researchers and therapists have listed standard definitions in the *Diagnostic and Statistical Manual of Mental Disorders (DSM)*. Continually kept up-to-date, this book helps doctors, psychiatrists, psychologists, and others who need to know the definition and diagnosis of depression. The current DSM definition lists nine symptoms of depression. At least five must persist for two or more weeks to qualify as depression.

It is extremely important that young people receive a correct diagnosis if they are depressed, so that they can then get the correct antidepressant medication and/or therapy. Unfortunately, too many young people are incorrectly diagnosed, often as schizophrenic. Young people who are depressed cannot get well on the type of medication used to treat schizophrenia.

Not FDA Approved for Children Under Twelve

Although the FDA has approved dozens of antidepressants to treat depression and other mental disorders in adults, it has not approved any antidepressant for use in children younger than age twelve. The FDA, however, does not limit the use of an antidepressant for other purposes. This means that a doctor can prescribe an antidepressant for a child or teen, even though the FDA has not specifically approved this use. Recently the FDA approved the testing of two antidepressants on depressed children.

No scientific proof exists that antidepressants help depressed children before puberty, the stage at which the reproductive organs become capable of functioning. This generally occurs

DSM Symptom of Depression	May Show Up As
Continually depressed mood	Blunted feelings, irritability, overreacting to frustrations and annoyances or opposition and anger, acting out in an antisocial way.
Markedly diminished interest or pleasure in all, or almost all activities	Loss of interest in school, falling grades, cutting classes. Does not participate in former hobbies, sports, clubs, or activities. Does not want to be with friends and friends pull away. Less interest in personal grooming. May look unkempt, frumpy, or may not brush hair or teeth.
Significant weight change without trying	Weight loss or gain. Loss of appetite or inability to enjoy food. Eating disorders such as anorexia or bulimia can be closely associated with depression.
Sleep problems during the night	Excessive sleeping or difficulty falling asleep, awakening too early, awakening often during the night.
Fatigue or energy loss, change in activity level	Low energy, fatigue, constant boredom. General slowing of thought, speech, and movement; appears sluggish. Or may become restless, jittery, or tense.
Negative feelings or thoughts	Persistent hopeless, negative, sad, empty, thoughts; often feels helpless, guilty, lonely, or worthless, coupled with feelings of isolation.
Diminished ability to think or make decisions	Inability to concentrate, remember things, or make decisions. Cannot focus on things such as a conversation, magazine article, or watch an entire television show.
Suicidal thoughts or talking about suicide attempts and plans	Reoccurring thoughts of death or suicide. Making final arrangements is another possible indicator. Teens might give away treasured personal possessions, such as a favorite book, record, or collection.

between ages thirteen and sixteen in boys and between twelve and fourteen in girls. No long-term information has been collected on the safety of antidepressants in children under age twelve.

To date, most antidepressant studies have been carried out on adults. Only one large study has been conducted that has shown that Prozac helps children and teens with major depression. Dr. Graham Emslie of the University of Texas Southwestern Medical School in Dallas followed ninety-six young people, ages eight to seventeen, with major depression. After eight weeks of treatment, over half (56 percent) of the young people were helped by Prozac. This study has not yet been published and it has not been reviewed by other specialists.[5]

Soon other studies will provide additional information. The manufacturer of Zoloft is gathering data on the use of this drug in treating children with OCD. Another manufacturer is running a study to see how its antidepressant, Paxil, works on ten- to eighteen-year-olds.

Unknown Risks

Some parents are concerned about the unknown long-term effects of antidepressants taken by young people, especially the newer SSRI antidepressants. Other parents are relieved to know that antidepressant medications are available to help young people with depression. Carolyn Sanger of the National Alliance for the Mentally Ill said that her son suffered from major depression when he was five. As he grew older, the episodes of depression continued. Finally, a doctor prescribed antidepressants for her son.[6]

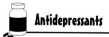

Despite the unknown long-term risks, Sanger opted to allow her son to take antidepressants. She explained that, "When your child talks of suicide, you're willing to risk that twenty years down the road there may be a serious side effect. I didn't think my son would live through high school." Her son took antidepressants every day for six years. The drugs, Sanger said, let him be a teen and enjoy life. Now in his early twenties, her son no longer takes antidepressants.[7]

Some researchers warn that it is too soon to determine the long-term effects of antidepressants on young people. Dr. Boris Birmaher, director of the Child and Adolescent Mood and Behavior Disorders Clinic at the University of Pittsburgh, stated his concern. "So far, we haven't seen any significant neurological [nerve] or growth problems, but sometimes it takes several years to discover them."[8]

One mother, Ruth Musicante, found that her young son developed an extreme reaction to an antidepressant after taking it for less than two weeks. Diagnosed at age six with depression and attention deficit disorder (ADD), her son took antidepressants for only ten days. His mother said that the antidepressant took away his impulse control, causing him to run in front of cars in the street and to attack a baby-sitter he has known for five years, drawing blood by scratching and biting him. The boy's doctor told his mother to stop giving her son the antidepressant, and after four days, the drug's effects wore off.[9]

Some critics say that taking SSRIs will cause symptoms of mania to appear, such as abnormally intense excitement and hyperactivity, in some depressed children and teens. This happens because it can be hard for a health professional to determine the type of depression present in a young person. The depression could be major depression or bipolar. If the depression is bipolar, then sometimes antidepressants can trigger mania.

That is what happened to Steven (not his real name). Beginning in his senior year of high school, he started to let his homework slide and brought home poor test scores. Before this, Steven was a very good student. One night Steven asked his mother to find out why he was having continual thoughts of death. "I feel like I can't get my mind off it. I'm too young to be having thoughts like these," he said.[10]

His mother was alarmed. To her, Steven seemed to be happy and to enjoy his friends and hobbies. She agreed to find a psychiatrist.[11] The psychiatrist who examined Steven said that he was depressed and that his death thoughts pointed to the possibility of Steven committing suicide. The doctor recommended an antidepressant but warned Steven and his mother about the potential for a manic episode. He detailed what a manic episode would be like: nervous energy, increasingly rapid thinking, and feeling out of control and uncomfortable.

Steven took the antidepressant for a few months but saw little change. Then one night, he felt anxious and told his mother that he could not sit still. He thought he might be getting manic. He was correct, and a doctor quickly prescribed a tranquilizer to control his mania. Steven had to stop taking his antidepressants.[12]

Eric's Success with Antidepressants

For several months, Eric (not his real name), age twelve, had complained of feeling tired, having little energy, and not sleeping well at night. His once hearty appetite had disappeared. The psychiatrist who examined him concluded that the boy was

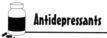

depressed and recommended both antidepressant medication and psychotherapy. Eric lived with his grandmother, and the two decided to first try therapy, since they felt uncomfortable with the idea of Eric taking a drug. They agreed to evaluate how the therapy was working after six weeks.[13]

After the six weeks were up, Eric said that the counseling had not helped much. The psychiatrist reexamined him and agreed. Eric's tests still showed that he was depressed. This time, after again hearing the pros and cons of antidepressant medication, Eric decided to try an antidepressant. Realizing that Eric was still uncomfortable with taking a drug, the psychiatrist suggested he make a simple rating chart of troubling symptoms such as "feeling tired all the time," "being bored a lot," and "not caring what happens."[14]

The psychiatrist started Eric on a low dose of the antidepressant to be sure he could tolerate it and that he could deal with any side effects. Since Eric was not bothered with many side effects, he took more of the antidepressant over the next two weeks until he was at the full-dose level prescribed by his doctor. He first noticed that he now slept through the night. Then his appetite perked up. After a month had gone by, he felt happier. The antidepressant continued to lessen Eric's depression over the next six weeks. Eric stayed on the antidepressant for five months, then tapered off. He has not had another bout of depression for three years.[15]

Antidepressants Help Prevent Suicide

A final result of severe depression is suicide. The number one risk factor in suicides is untreated depression.[16] Suicides among

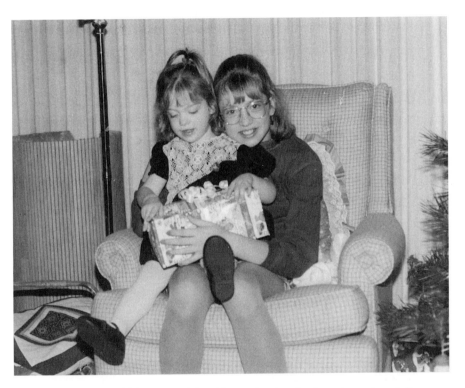

Before the 1980s, mental health professionals thought only adults developed severe depression. They have since learned that young people can also have this mental illness. It is treatable with antidepressants and therapy.

young people have increased dramatically. Since the 1980s, the suicide rate for ten- to fourteen-year-olds has risen 120 percent and the rate for fifteen- to nineteen-year-olds has risen by 28.3 percent.[17] Suicide is the third leading cause of death for fifteen- to twenty-four-year-olds, and the sixth leading cause of death for five- to fourteen-year-olds.[18] That translates into two thousand teen suicides each year in the United States.[19] Many of these suicides could be prevented if these young people were to receive treatment with antidepressant medication and/or psychotherapy.

Researchers estimate that two hundred fifty thousand children and teens try to kill themselves every year. Many suicides go unreported, however, so that figure could actually be twice as high.[20] Although the suicide rate for teens is much higher than it is for children, researchers have reported that suicides have increased among younger children.[21] Researchers have reported that children as young as five with untreated depression have committed suicide.

These statistics on teen suicide are staggering, but treatment for depression with antidepressant medications offers great hope. Antidepressants lift depression and the feelings and thoughts of hopelessness, death, dying, and suicide.

At age sixteen, Emmy (not her real name) nearly became another teen suicide statistic. Before her depression took control, Emmy juggled a busy schedule. She maintained a *B-plus* grade average, held a part-time job, and was on her school's swim team. She wanted more from herself, though—she wanted to be an *A* student. But no matter how hard she studied, she could not raise her grades any higher.[22]

After a while, she stopped caring about her grades and working so hard. "Nothing special happened; I just shut down. I felt

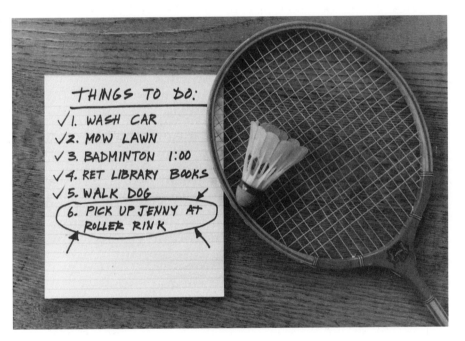

When prescribed by a doctor, antidepressants can help depressed teens feel restored to their normal selves.

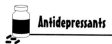

so alone, like I was living in a bubble and couldn't punch my way out," she remembered.[23]

She began hearing a constant buzzing in her head and had trouble concentrating and having enough energy to even eat. Emmy recalled, "I didn't want to do anything except lie on my bed and listen to tapes. When my friends called, I didn't feel like talking to them. I knew they were getting mad, and sometimes I'd try to talk on the phone, but I couldn't push the words up out of my throat."[24]

Finally, Emmy decided life was not worth living and decided to commit suicide. She took an overdose of pills. Luckily, she was rushed to a hospital and survived. While recovering at the hospital, Emmy's doctor diagnosed her severe depression and started her on antidepressant medication. The drug worked, and as the months went by, Emmy regained her energy and zest for life. After six months, she went off the antidepressant and is once more planning her future.[25]

The Future of Antidepressants and Young People

Doctors prescribe the tricyclic antidepressants most often for young people with depression. That is because doctors have studied these drugs for over thirty years and understand their uses and side effects. Doctors seldom recommend MAOIs for young people. Their many food interactions are troublesome to deal with for children and teens.

Doctors are also prescribing the SSRIs more and more often for young people. Many mental health professionals say that these drugs have fewer side effects than the older tricyclic antidepressants. Due to the higher risk of serious side effects, doctors must monitor the heart or blood levels of a child or teen on tricyclic antidepressants. Such costly, ongoing laboratory tests are not needed for young people on the SSRIs.

Prozac often ranks high as the doctor's choice when prescribing an antidepressant for a young person today. This is because Prozac is taken only once a day, unlike the older tricyclic antidepressants, which are often taken two or more times a day. This means a teen is less likely to forget to take it. Also, a young person cannot overdose and die from taking too much Prozac or any of the other SSRI antidepressants.

Questions for Discussion

1. Sometimes it is hard to ask for help. Suggest some ways a friend might ask for help when needed.

2. Over the last couple of months, you have noticed that a friend has become moody and irritable. Now this friend tells you about a suicide plan but asks that you not tell anyone. What would you do?

3. Some people feel blue during the holidays. Suggest ways to help prevent the holiday blues.

5

Cyclic Antidepressants

Cyclic antidepressants are divided into two groups. The older ones are called tricyclic antidepressants (TCAs) because of their similar chemical structure of three interlocking carbon rings. They have been the "cornerstone of drug therapy for depression" for over thirty-five years, because they have proven extremely effective in treating depression.[1] They are also the largest class or group of antidepressant drugs. Some of the better known ones include Tofranil (imipramine), Elavil (amitriptyline), and Pamelor (Nortriptyline). Newer cyclics have different numbers of carbon rings. They include ones such as Desyrel™ (trazadone) and Wellbutrin™ (bupropion).

Who Can Take TCAs

Many doctors prescribe TCAs because of their long history of use compared to the much more recent SSRIs and SNRIs. Doctors are also familiar with their side effects. Doctors can safely prescribe TCAs for young people and pregnant women. The SSRIs are still too new to determine if they would harm a developing baby. Mothers who are nursing their babies cannot take TCAs, however, because the medication is passed on to the baby through the breast milk.

People with a history of heart disease should use TCAs carefully or avoid them altogether because these drugs can create heart problems.[2] Individuals may also need to stay away from TCAs if they are on other drugs that can interact with them. Examples of these drugs include: thyroid supplements, high blood pressure medications, oral contraceptives (birth control pills), some sleeping medications, diuretics (water pills), antihistamines, aspirin, vitamin C, alcohol, and tobacco. The combination of a TCA and alcohol is particularly dangerous. This is because the two drugs will interact and magnify the TCA's effects in unpredictable ways.

Those who wear soft contact lenses may also find that they cannot take TCAs. That is because these medications tend to decrease the normal level of tears. By drying the eyes so much, thick secretions can build up on the contact lenses, causing itching and grittiness. To deal with this problem, the doctor can reduce the dosage of the antidepressant, try a different antidepressant, or prescribe the use of eye drops.

What It Feels Like to Take Cyclics

People taking cyclic antidepressants do not get high. They seldom are aware of being on a medication, except that their depressive symptoms become less intense and they function better. The benefits of cyclics can take several weeks to become apparent. Sometimes the changes are not obvious. The person may be slow to realize the depression is lifting. People who take cyclic antidepressants do not escape, ignore, or become numb to their problems.[3]

One of the first improvements people notice when taking cyclics is improved sleep. They will get more restful sleep, often with fewer nightmares. The drug also increases energy and ability to concentrate and perks up decreased appetites. Negative thinking and sadness lifts.

Side Effects

Every person differs in the degree and type of side effects he or she experiences with cyclic antidepressants. Some people never have any side effects. The number of possible side effects with TCAs vary, depending on the medication and the person. Because of this kind of variation in side effects, one TCA might be highly desirable for one person and not recommended for another.

"Youngsters often experience fewer troublesome side effects than adults do," noted Dr. Lawrence L. Kerns, a psychiatrist specializing in childhood depression.[4] However, these people can often safely take lower doses of antidepressants and find relief from their depression.

TCAs can produce some troubling side effects. Some side effects disappear quickly, while others may remain for the length

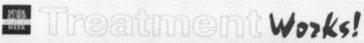

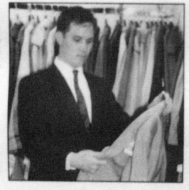
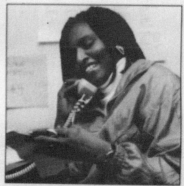
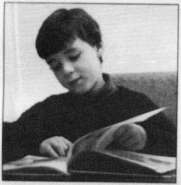
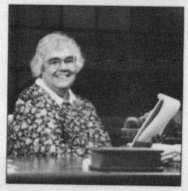

MENTAL ILLNESS AWARENESS WEEK

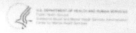

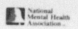

Although the exact causes of depression are still debated, the symptoms are well established. The disorder can be treated with antidepressants and psychotherapy.

of treatment. As the body adjusts to the drug, temporary side effects can occur during the first month or two of starting a TCA. Although it may be tempting to stop taking the drug, over time, the side effects lessen or disappear and the benefits begin to appear.

Common Side Effects of Tricyclic Antidepressants

At the start of treatment:

- *Feeling restless or anxious*
- *Night sweats*
- *Trouble concentrating*
- *Trouble falling asleep or disturbed sleep*

These side effects often disappear after two or three weeks.

Ongoing:

- *Dry mouth or eyes*
- *Constipation*
- *Drowsiness*
- *Increased sweating*
- *Lightheadedness or dizziness, especially when rising from a sitting or lying position*
- *Muscle twitches, weakness*
- *Nausea*
- *Sensitivity to bright light*
- *Unpleasant taste in the mouth*
- *Weight gain and sugar craving*

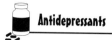

Serious side effects—consult a doctor:

- *Blurred vision or eye pain*
- *Confusion, nightmares, hallucinations*
- *Fainting, tremors*
- *Seizures, especially if person has a prior head injury or history of seizures*
- *Irregular or too rapid heart beat*
- *Shakiness*
- *Skin rash, hives, swelling of face or tongue*
- *Sore throat and fever*
- *Trouble urinating*

Dealing with the Side Effects of TCAs

People usually tolerate the side effects of TCAs or develop simple coping methods. For example, chewing sugarless gum, sucking on sugarless hard candy, or drinking sips of water regularly, helps dry mouth. If dry mouth is especially troublesome, the doctor can prescribe a medication that increases the flow of saliva. Low levels of saliva can promote tooth decay and gum problems, so people who take TCAs need to get regular dental care.

Drinking more water and adding fiber to your diet by eating plenty of whole grains, fruits, and vegetables helps constipation. Exercise helps, too. If needed, the doctor can prescribe a laxative or switch the person to a different antidepressant. A queasy stomach can be avoided by taking the antidepressant with food. Some people get drowsy when they begin taking a TCA. It is best if they do not drive or operate heavy equipment during this period. This usually passes within two to three weeks.

Weight gain is also a common side effect of many TCAs, although no one knows why. If weight gain occurs, perhaps switching to a different antidepressant will tame the appetite. However, a different antidepressant may not work in dealing with the depression. If the current antidepressant is relieving depression, then the person will need to decide if losing the weight is possible, or if they can live with it.

It takes several weeks of continual use of TCAs to determine if the side effects are tolerable.[5] If the side effects are unacceptable or serious, the doctor may try another antidepressant. It is difficult to predict which antidepressant and dosage level will work the best for each person.

Precautions

TCAs tend to slow the heart rate. Since this can cause irregular heart rate or heart block, TCAs are generally not recommended for people with preexisting heart conditions. These drugs can also cause seizures for people with a history of seizures.[6]

Overdoses of TCAs can be life-threatening. According to Elliot Gelwan at Harvard Medical School, TCAs are the leading cause of death by drug overdose in the United States.[7]

People should not increase the dose of their cyclic antidepressant without consulting their doctor. Taking too much of a cyclic antidepressant will overstimulate the central nervous system. This can result in seizures, heart problems, or even death. People have died from as little as 500 mg of amitriptyline or imipramine; the usual doses for both drugs are 100 to 300 mg. Other deaths have occurred when people took a one-to two-week supply at one time.[8]

An overdose of tricyclic antidepressants requires immediate medical attention. Symptoms of an overdose of tricyclic antidepressants develop within an hour. They may start with rapid heartbeat, dilated or enlarged pupils, flushed face, and agitation. If left untreated, the person can become confused, have seizures, and develop an irregular heartbeat. Finally, the heart stops and death occurs.

Treatment Plan

The prescribing doctor will develop a treatment plan for each person taking antidepressants. The tricyclic is usually started at a low dose to determine if the person can tolerate it. This also allows the body to slowly adjust to the tricyclic's effects. Then the dose is increased every two to four days until it is at the correct daily dose. This can take from one to three weeks. The dosage varies depending on the drug.

Some people divide their TCA dose over two to four times a day. Because TCAs are long lasting, other people take their whole dose at bedtime. This way, side effects peak overnight and any sedating effects will not be noticed the next day. However, if the person wakes up tired, the dose can be taken after dinner or divided into two or more portions and taken at different times of the day.

To be effective, TCAs must be taken every day. People cannot use them as needed, such as when they feel really low. To determine if the tricyclic antidepressant will lift depression, the person must stay on it for several weeks. If no or only partial improvement results, the doctor may increase the dosage level or

#1 CAUSE OF SUICIDE
UNTREATED
DEPRESSION
SA\VE SUICIDE AWARENESS VOICES OF EDUCATION

People with untreated mental illnesses, such as depression, have higher suicide rates than those who do not have such mental disorders.

switch to a different cyclic or different class of antidepressant. People should contact their doctor or pharmacist with questions about their tricyclic antidepressant.

Length of Treatment

If they respond well, people usually are taken off their tricyclic antidepressants after six to twelve months.[9] Doctors advise people who are going off of tricyclics to gradually taper off over two to three weeks. Otherwise, depressive symptoms could recur, especially if the drug is stopped too soon. Withdrawal symptoms can be tough to deal with. Chills, restlessness, fatigue, vomiting, stuffy nose or other cold symptoms, nausea, headaches, sleeping problems, and nightmares, and muscle aches and pains are all possible side effects.

People who have had several depressive episodes may elect to

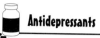

stay on tricyclic antidepressants for life. According to the Agency for Health Care Policy and Research, people who have had three episodes of major depression have a 90 percent chance of having another. The World Health Organization (WHO) recommends lifelong treatment with cyclic antidepressants for people who have had two depressive episodes within a five-year period.[10]

Questions for Discussion

1. Someday, scientists hope to develop a test to determine genetic predisposition to depression. Can you see any potential conflicts in the use of such a test?

2. Unhappiness stems naturally from many situations and offers people a chance to examine themselves and make changes. Some people use alcohol and other drugs to cover up their unhappiness. In the long run, though, this does not work. Why?

3. People who attempt suicide are often under a great deal of stress. Suggest some ways to reduce stress.

6

MAOIs

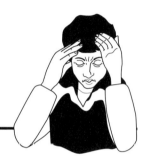

Monoamine oxidase inhibitors (MAOIs) are powerful antidepressants that can produce great improvements for those with depression. However, they can also trigger severe side effects and require a special diet. Because of this, MAOIs are not usually a doctor's first choice.

If people avoid the restricted foods, beverages, and medications, however, there is little chance of serious side effects from MAOIs. Dr. Donald L. Klein has found that MAOIs are "very useful" and "are often effective when other antidepressants are not."[1] Dr. Mark S. Gold agrees. "Generally . . . MAOIs are safe and effective and have little potential for abuse or overdose."[2]

In the early 1980s, Dick Cavett, television host and actor, could no longer cope with his chronic depression. He had felt that his "brain was 'broken'" and that "Everything seemed to be growing gray. All the things that used to give me pleasure suddenly weren't worth the effort."[3]

Cavett stayed in a hospital for five weeks, waiting for his MAOI to take effect. The MAOI, which he has since taken every day for over a decade, has worked. It restored his zest for life and his wit, humor, and speaking abilities. After years of MAOI treatment, his depression, said Cavett, is "absolutely chemical."[4]

What It Feels Like to Take MAOIs

As with the tricyclics, people taking MAOIs do not get high or addicted. They seldom are aware of being on a medication, except that their depressive symptoms become less intense and they function better. The benefits of MAOIs generally take several weeks to occur.[5] Sometimes the changes are not obvious. It may take a while for the person to realize that the depression is lifting.

Who Can Take MAIOs?

If someone does not respond to the tricyclic antidepressants, doctors sometimes try MAOIs next. Some research suggests that MAOIs can help those with chronic depression. They can also be used by people with heart disease.

MAOIs also work particularly well for people with atypical depression. People with atypical depression can enjoy life, but they oversleep and overeat, especially sweets. Their depression is chronic—long-lasting with the potential for frequent recurrence—and generally starts in their teens, with a lack of interest, energy, and get-up-and-go. Sometimes they have panic attacks or intense phobias.

Barbara (not her real name) sought help for her depression, which had followed her since childhood. She complained of constant tiredness, often overslept for hours, and spent a lot of time resting in bed. She was only ten pounds overweight but felt fat. Barbara enjoyed a good party and could have fun. However, she could not handle rejection, which made her angry and depressed. She also complained of recurring panic attacks.[6]

When her doctor prescribed a cyclic antidepressant, Barbara's depression did not lift. She then tried an MAOI, and responded well. She lost weight, felt peppy, and got along better with her husband. Her panic attacks disappeared. She decided to stop taking the drug after six months, but her symptoms returned. After resuming her regular dosage, she felt like herself again.[7]

MAOIs have a high potential for interacting with other drugs and certain foods. This can limit their use in people who are taking other medications or are unable to restrict their diet.

Side Effects

MAOIs produce some of the same side effects as the tricyclic antidepressants. Dizziness when changing position and rapid heartbeat are common. Other side effects include sleeping problems, dizziness, dry mouth, headache, rash, weakness, restlessness, fatigue, constipation, and weight gain. Sometimes fluid is retained in the fingers and ankles. These side effects generally lessen or disappear with continued use. The doctor may also decrease the dose to lessen the side effects.

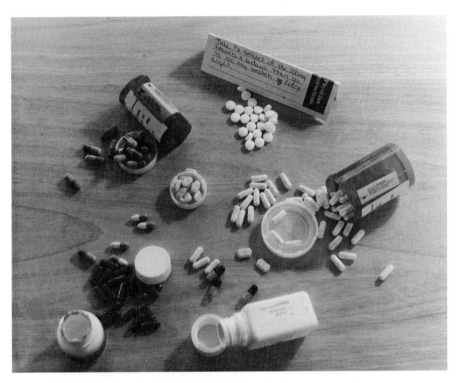

Antidepressants provide effective treatment for depression. However, any drug powerful enough to alter moods can also produce unwanted side effects.

According to Dr. Mark S. Gold at the University of Florida College of Medicine, in some people, MAOIs can cause euphoria or a feeling of being high. Also, MAOIs sometimes promote hyperactivity or excess activity in those with bipolar disorder.

Precautions

MAOIs can produce dangerously high blood pressure if they react with the amino acid tyramine. Tyramine occurs naturally in many foods and helps regulate blood pressure. However, MAOIs stop enzymes in the body from breaking down tyramine. High protein food snacks that have been aged, ripened, fermented, pickled, or smoked can contain a lot of tyramine.

To safely take an MAOI a person must completely avoid these foods and certain medications. Even eating a small amount of banned food could cause a negative interaction with an MAOI. Here is why. Under ordinary cicumstances, tyramine moves into the brain after a person eats sausage or aged cheese. Enzymes break down the tyramine and blood pressure remains normal. The MAOI, however, prevents the enzymes from working, so the tyramine level stays too high and blood pressure skyrockets.

If someone is taking an MAOI and eats a banned food, several hours will usually pass before the person suffers any reaction. This is sometimes known as the "cheese reaction."[8] Symptoms of the reaction can include a headache, racing or pounding heart, visual problems, neck pain or stiffness, confusion, nausea, fatigue, vomiting, and fainting. The person may not have any warning that blood pressure has zoomed. With or without any accompanying warnings, the result of such high blood pressure is

Foods and Beverages to Avoid if Taking an MAOI

- ✔ Ale
- ✔ Anchovies
- ✔ Avocado
- ✔ Bean curd or tofu
- ✔ **Beans** *(broad beans, fresh or dried, such as fava beans, lima beans, and green beans)*
- ✔ **Beer** *(including alcohol-free and reduced-alcohol products)*
- ✔ Caviar
- ✔ **Cheese** *(especially strong or aged cheese such as cheddar—cottage cheese and cream cheese are OK)*
- ✔ **Chocolate** *(in large amounts)*
- ✔ **Dry sausage** *(including all salamis and pepperoni)*
- ✔ Figs
- ✔ **Fish** *(smoked, fermented, pickled, or aged)*
- ✔ Ginseng
- ✔ **Liver** *(especially chicken and beef liver)*

- ✔ Meat tenderizers or extracts
- ✔ Over-ripe bananas
- ✔ Pea pods
- ✔ Pizza
- ✔ Protein dietary supplements
- ✔ Sauerkraut
- ✔ Shrimp paste
- ✔ **Smoked, pickled, fermented, or other processed meats, fish, or soy products** *(includes lunch meats, sausages, and soy sauce)*
- ✔ **Soups** *(canned and instant soup powders)*
- ✔ Sour cream
- ✔ **Wine** *(including alcohol-free and reduced-alcohol wine products)*
- ✔ **Yeast extracts** *(such as yeast vitamin supplements)*
- ✔ Yogurt

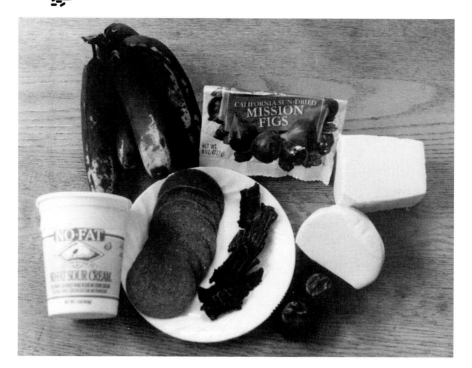

To avoid a life-threatening interaction, people on MAOIs must follow a restricted diet and avoid such foods as cheese, chocolate, beef jerky, salami, sour cream, bananas, and figs.

serious—severe headache, seizures, stroke, or even death can occur.[9]

If someone on an MAOI uses nose drops, cold remedies, or other banned medication, these same reactions can occur. These medications are chemically similar to tyramine. They cannot be broken down when someone is taking an MAOI. People who take MAOIs need to notify their doctor of all other medications they are taking—including non-presription medications. Some doctors suggest that people try out the restricted diet for a few days or a week before taking the drug. This helps determine if a person can successfully adapt to such a changed lifestyle.

Managing Interactions

Some doctors give people taking MAOIs a blood-pressure medication to carry with them at all times. A headache is often the first sign of a high blood pressure reaction with an MAOI. If a headache develops, the person should take the medication with them and get to an emergency room. Hospital staff will check the blood pressure and begin treatment to bring down high blood pressure.

MAOIs generally work quickly with no serious side effects. However, if someone already gets a lot of headaches, MAOIs are not a good antidepressant choice.

MAOI overdoses can be deadly. People should not increase their dose of MAOIs without consulting their doctor. Taking too much can lead to seizures, confusion, coma, breathing difficulties, shock, or heart problems.

Treatment Plan

The prescribing doctor will develop an individual treatment plan for each person. The MAOI is generally started at a low dose to determine if the person can tolerate it. This also allows the body to slowly adjust to the MAOIs effects. Then the dose is increased rapidly. People should contact their doctor or pharmacist if they have any questions about their MAOI.

MAOIs are usually taken two or three times during the day. They are not generally taken at bedtime because they tend to cause insomnia. MAOIs must be taken every day. People cannot use

Drugs to Avoid if Taking an MAOI

✔ Anesthesia

✔ Antiasthma
 medications

✔ Antihistamines

✔ Antiparkinsonian
 medications

✔ Appetite suppressants

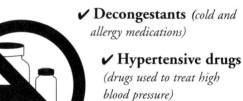

✔ Decongestants *(cold and
 allergy medications)*

✔ **Hypertensive drugs**
 *(drugs used to treat high
 blood pressure)*

✔ Insulin

✔ Sedatives

✔ Tricyclic antidepressants

them as needed such as when they feel really low. To determine if an MAOI will work, the person must stay on it for several weeks. If no or only partial improvement results, the doctor may increase the dosage or switch to a different MAOI or different class of antidepressant.

When switching from another antidepressant class, such as the tricyclic to an MAOI, the person must not take any antidepressant for seven to ten days. If switching from an MAOI to an antidepressant of another class, such as a tricyclic, allow a washout period of fourteen days when no antidepressants of any kind are taken. This washout period allows the body to washout or remove any of the first antidepressant.[10]

Doctors advise not to stop taking an MAOI abruptly. Instead, the person needs to taper off the MAOI over several weeks to reduce withdrawal symptoms. If someone suddenly stops taking an MAOI or stops taking the MAOI too soon, another depressive episode can flare up.

Promising MAOIs on the Horizon

Although not yet available in the United States, a new class of MAOIs, sometimes called reversible MAOIs, has been developed recently. One such drug does not require a special diet. Currently, doctors in Switzerland can prescribe it. Dr. Donald F. Klein has predicted that these new antidepressants "will prove very popular and useful" when they come to the United States.[11]

Questions for Discussion

1. Staying healthy is important for all of us because it affects how we feel about ourselves. What are some of the ways that you maintain your health?

2. Talking to someone you trust is one way to sort out your emotions and feelings. Can you think of other ways?

3. Studies done by the National Institute of Mental Health find that the number of people suffering from depression has increased since 1970. What are some possible reasons for this increase?

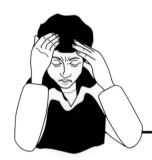

7

SSRIs and SNRIs

Selective Serotonin Reuptake Inhibitors (SSRIs) and Serotonin Nonselective Reuptake Inhibitors (SNRIs) are the newest classes of antidepressants. Although chemically different from the tricyclics and MAOIs, these newer drugs are just as effective. Three SSRIs and two SNRIs are sold by prescription in the United States. The SSRIs include Prozac (fluoxetine), Zoloft (sertaline), and Paxil (paroxetine). The SNRIs are Effexor (venlafaxine) and Serzone™ (nefazodone).

Transforming Drugs?

These newer antidepressants offer great help in treating depression, but they do not work any quicker than other classes of antidepressants. Some of their side effects are less troublesome, but they have their own set of side effects and problems. One misconception is the idea that antidepressants transform or change someone's personality. This is simply not true.

Ron's (not his real name) use of an antidepressant seemed to transform him into a different teen. During his school years, Ron stayed to himself and worked on his computer. During high school, he totally withdrew from people. He stopped cleaning himself and wore dirty clothes. Even his computer no longer held his attention. Finally, Ron was diagnosed with depression and began taking an antidepressant. Ron's energy level surged, he kept himself clean and well groomed, and he became friends with some of his classmates. He even got a girlfriend.

Now his doctor puzzled over what to do. Should Ron stay on the antidepressant and continue as the "improved" Ron? Or, because he was no longer depressed, should Ron go off the antidepressant and perhaps return to his quiet, withdrawn self? Had the antidepressant uncovered the "real" Ron, one that had been chronically depressed? Or was this new Ron a false self?[1] The antidepressant did not change Ron's personality. It did, however, help him recover from his episode of depression.

All antidepressants, including the SSRIs and SNRIs, are designed to relieve the symptoms of depression. They only work for people who have depression. However, some doctors call them "mood brighteners" because they seem to enhance life for healthy, normal people such as Tess.

Tess (not her real name) was a successful businessperson, but said she was unhappy and lacked energy. Her doctor prescribed Prozac and within two weeks, Tess reported that she no longer felt tired. Instead, she felt rested and hopeful. Soon she began dating and enjoyed making new friends. Tess stayed on Prozac for nine months, then stopped taking the drug. But after eight months, she asked to go back on the antidepressant because she felt "she was slipping" and was no longer her improved self.[2]

Did Prozac turn Tess into a new or improved person? Are the SSRIs and SNRIs mood brighteners or wonder drugs? No, say the experts. The evidence that these drugs make people "better than well" is anecdotal evidence, that is one person's or one doctor's word or claim.[3] Experts say that these drugs can help mildly depressed people like Tess shed their depression and regain their normal personalities.[4]

Dr. Philip Gold, a researcher at the National Institute of Mental Health summed up the current research on this issue. People who are on an even keel "do not respond to antidepressants. The idea that healthy people who take Prozac feel better is absolutely ridiculous."[5]

More Controversy

After its introduction in 1988, Prozac began receiving a lot of media attention. Why? Prozac was the first new class of antidepressants, the SSRIs, created since the 1950s. Also, because of its selective action on only one neurotransmitter, serotonin, people who take Prozac and the other SSRIs often do not experience many of the TCAs' annoying side effects such as dry eyes and mouth. Americans have also had an increased awareness of depression and that this disease can be treated with antidepressant medication.

This awareness is due, to a great degree, to various federal and national groups that sponsor educational programs about

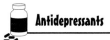

depression and its treatment. One of these groups is the Depression, Awareness, Recognition, and Treatment (DART) program, sponsored by the National Institute of Mental Health. Also, the media has played up the false idea that Prozac can transform personalities. All these factors swept Prozac into center stage as a miracle drug for depression.

However, in mid-September 1989, Prozac plunged into negative publicity. Newspapers reported that an unemployed printer from Louisville, Kentucky, had randomly shot twenty people, killing eight and wounding twelve at his former print shop. He then shot and killed himself. He had been taking Prozac. Later, an article in the *Wall Street Journal* reported that before taking Prozac, this man had tried to commit suicide twelve times, owned many guns, and was a good shot.

A few months later, in November 1989, the Church of Scientology attacked Prozac. This group has stated that its goal is to "remove psychiatry completely from the world and put Scientology in its place as the foremost mental-health therapy."[6] The Scientologists spent millions of dollars on an anti-Prozac campaign, saying that the drug causes people to become suicidal and commit murders.[7]

Then Dr. Martin Teicher, a Harvard Medical School psychiatrist, published a paper that described six depressed people, who while taking Prozac, had become preoccupied with suicidal thoughts. The Scientiologists used this report in their campaign, although they ignored three important facts:

> *(1) Four of the six were on other powerful medications besides Prozac.*

(2) Five of the six had thought about or attempted suicide in the past.

(3) Other patients of Dr. Teicher's had benefited from Prozac, and had no suicidal thoughts.[8]

The turning point came in October 1990 when the Citizens Commission on Human Rights, a group founded by the Church of Scientology, asked the FDA to ban Prozac. The FDA regulates prescription medications. Meanwhile people began suing Eli Lilly and Company, the makers of Prozac. They said that the antidepressant had plunged them into suicidal or violent action.

After studying the facts, the FDA refused to ban Prozac. An FDA panel found "no credible evidence" that linked the drug and violent behavior.[9] To date, no proof exists that Prozac causes violent, hostile, or suicidal behavior. Many of those suing have had histories of violence or suicide attempts or other long-term major medical or emotional problems. The courts have dismissed all lawsuits against the makers of Prozac.

The authors of *The Essential Guide to Prescription Drugs* sum up the current research on this issue. "Suicidal thinking may emerge during treatment with any antidepressant. Recent reports establish that some patients who become suicidal while taking one antidepressant can be switched to fluoxetine [Prozac] and experience cessation [an end to] suicidal thinking and satisfactory relief of depression."[10] Today, all the SSRIs are accepted and useful antidepressant medications.

Who Can Take SSRIs and SNRIs

SSRIs are often prescribed for elderly people. The SSRIs tend to have milder side effects, which can be handled by older people.

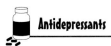

However, older people may not deal well with the most common side effects of these drugs such as nausea and diarrhea.

The SSRIs are a good choice for people with heart conditions. Compared to TCAs, they cause fewer heart problems. Also, SSRIs are less likely to cause low blood pressure.

People with a kidney or liver disease should not take SSRIs. These drugs are metabolized or broken down in the liver and moved to the kidneys. If these organs are not working well, high levels of the SSRIs can build up in the body. SSRIs cannot be taken by people with severe allergies. Those people who break out in a rash or hives after starting SSRI treatment also cannot continue to take these drugs.

What It Feels Like to Take SSRIs and SNRIs

People taking SSRIs and SNRIs do not get high. They seldom are aware of being on a medication, except that their depressive symptoms become less intense and they function better. The benefits of SSRIs and SNRIs can take several weeks to become apparent. Some people have reported positive results within a few days or weeks after starting an SSRI. Sometimes the changes are not obvious. It may take a while before the person realizes the depression is lifting.[11]

One of the first improvements people notice when taking an SSRI or SNRI is improved sleep. They get more restful sleep, often with fewer nightmares. The drug also increases energy and ability to concentrate and perks up decreased appetites. Negative thinking, anxiety, and sadness lifts.

Mary (not her real name) had long "felt like a misfit, as though I were living in a world created for other people. Often I

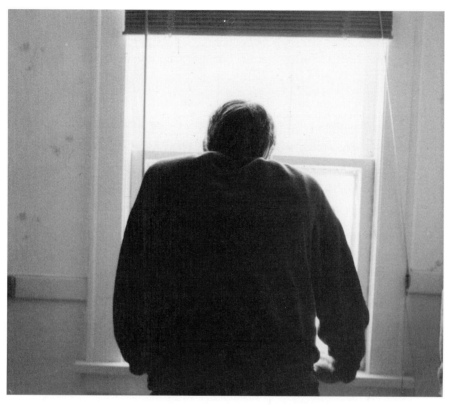

People who take antidepressants will still experience sadness and loneliness, but they will not stay down for extended periods of time.

told those close to me that maybe I didn't belong on this planet." After getting laid off from her job, she became depressed and suicidal. Luckily, she found a psychiatrist who carefully listened to her and suggested she take Zoloft. To Mary's relief, she found that "Zoloft has freed me from instability. For the first time in my conscious memory, I'm not at the mercy of my own mood swings."[12]

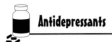

Ann (not her real name) began using Prozac in 1992 after having bouts of depression. She recalled, "I felt like a new person. It became easier to function, and I believe I became a more effective person overall."[13] About a year later, Ann started having anxiety and severe depression. Since the Prozac™ seemed to cause these symptoms, she stopped taking it. She tried a cyclic antidepressant, but the drug triggered a seizure, vomiting, headaches, and confusion.

Ann next tried an SNRI. Outside of headaches and nausea, she has responded well to this antidepressant. She has more energy and feels better about herself. Ann summed up, "The medication seems to have helped stabilize my mood, and I am hopeful that this will continue."[14]

Side Effects

Every person differs in the degree and types of side effects they experience with SSRIs and SNRIs. Some people never get any side effects. Others experience many side effects. Although it may be tempting to stop taking the drug if uncomfortable side effects occur, these side effects usually lessen or disappear within days or weeks. If not, the doctor will adjust the dose or have the person take the medication at a different time of day.

During the first couple weeks of taking Paxil, Sue (not her real name) had nausea, diarrhea, and dry mouth. As she continued on the drug, the effects disappeared. Sue now finds, "The medication has put me on an even keel. I can handle close to anything now. I am much happier, don't yell constantly, can focus now."[15]

Sometimes people can have serious reactions to SSRIs. Donna (not her real name) started taking Paxil on a Friday. By

Sunday, her tongue was partially numb and she had trouble urinating. The next day, she could not taste food. Over the next couple days, as she continued to take Paxil on the advice of her doctor, she often lost her balance while standing or walking, completely lost her appetite, and her mouth felt unusually dry. Finally, Donna lost all sense of hot and cold and became semiconscious from heat exhaustion. She was rushed to the emergency room, where the staff found her blood pressure much too high and her breathing forced and irregular. She immediately stopped taking Paxil. Two days later, she could feel some parts of her body responding normally.[16]

Unlike TCAs, SSRIs target only the system that regulates mood. This means that the SSRIs often do not cause some of the side effects common to the TCAs such as dry mouth and eyes, blurry vision, and changed heart function. The TCAs affect several of the body's chemical systems, including the one that regulates mood.

Side Effects of SSRI and SNRI Antidepressants

- *Diarrhea or constipation*
- *Feeling jittery or agitated*
- *Headaches*
- *Nausea*
- *Sexual problems*
- *Sleeping problems, such as insomnia or drowsiness*
- *Tremors*
- *Vivid dreams or intense nightmares*
- *Weight loss or gain*

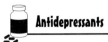

Serious side effects—consult a doctor:

- *Fever*

- *Joint swelling*

- *Seizures*

- *Skin rash, hives*

- *Sore throat and fever*

- *Swollen lymph glands*

- *Weakness*

Precautions

Since SSRIs and SNRIs have not been used much in people with heart, liver, or kidney conditions, doctors must monitor their use in people with these conditions. Use of these drugs must also be closely watched in people with histories of seizures. Unlike cyclic and MAOI antidepressants, overdoses of SSRIs and SNRIs are safer since the risk of harm to the heart or nervous system is small.[17]

SSRIs can interact with MAOIs and other medications. However, few researchers have studied the possible drug interactions of these antidepressants and do not know all of the possible harmful combinations. Mothers who are breast feeding babies cannot take SSRIs because these antidepressants are passed on to the baby through the breast milk. The FDA has not approved the use of SSRIs and SNRIs in young people with depression, but researchers are performing these types of studies now.

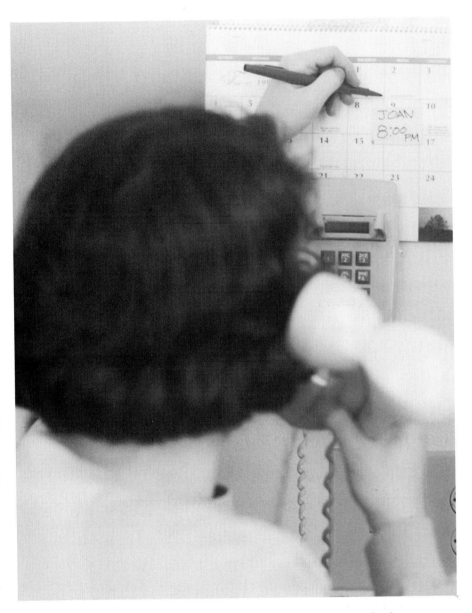

Antidepressants bring nerve transmissions in the brain back into balance. This restores normal moods, so that people can again take an interest in life.

Treatment Plan

Doctors recommend that people take SSRIs and SNRIs with food to lessen nausea. The dosage of SSRIs and SNRIs varies depending on the particular drug. SSRIs are generally taken once a day. If the dose of Prozac is more than 20 mg per day, people usually take it in divided doses twice a day. The SNRIs are taken in divided doses, usually two or three times during the day. People should contact their doctor or pharmacist with questions about their antidepressant.

Doctors have noticed that the easier a medication is to take, the more likely it is that people will take it. All of the SSRIs can be taken only once a day, which increases the odds that people will remember to take it. Many take their SSRI in the morning, with breakfast. If people experience troubling side effects such as sleeping problems or a feeling of hyperactivity, they can try taking the dose twice a day or take the full dose at bedtime.

To be effective, antidepressants must be taken every day. People cannot use them as needed, such as when they feel really low. To determine if the SSRIs or SNRIs will lift the depression, the person must stay on it for several weeks. If no or only partial improvement results, the doctor can increase the dosage or switch to a different antidepressant medication.

If they respond well, many people stop taking their antidepressants after six to twelve months. The SNRIs and sometimes the SSRIs cause withdrawal symptoms including weakness, dizziness, headaches, insomnia, nausea, and nervousness. To reduce withdrawal symptoms, people usually taper off these antidepressants over several weeks.

People who have had recurring depression can elect to stay on antidepressants for life to prevent another episode. Because the older tricyclic antidepressants have been used for over thirty years, researchers know they are safe for long-term use. As newer drugs, SSRIs and SNRIs have no long-term safety track record, so doctors advise caution.

Norah (not her real name) managed to make it through a depressive episode without treatment. Not wanting a repeat, she started on Prozac. At first Norah noticed only side effects: dry mouth, feeling like she was getting a cold, nausea, loss of appetite, and weight loss. A month later, her family saw a happier, more relaxed Norah. She now says Prozac saved her life. "I'll take Prozac until the day I die, if it will keep my brain functioning correctly. Sometimes I have to remind myself that it's a chemical problem in my brain. That it's not me, or who I am."[18]

Success Rates

With all of the success stories printed about Prozac, Paxil, and Zoloft, researchers have run studies to see if the media coverage is exaggerated. They have found that these newer drugs have the same success rate as the older TCAs. For example, researchers at the State University of New York examined thirteen published studies of antidepressants. About two-thirds of people taking Prozac or other antidepressants were helped. When compared to the other antidepressants, Prozac's success rate was about the same.

This agrees with the findings of the United States Agency for Health Care Policy and Research. It reported that no one antidepressant medication is clearly more effective than another in relieving depression.[19] It also has stated that no single antidepressant medication works for all people.[20]

Questions for Discussion

1. Any new drug, including an antidepressant, undergoes a decade or more of testing before the Food and Drug Administration can approve it for use in the United States. Do you think all of this testing is necessary? Why? Why not?

2. How would you feel if a parent or sibling was hospitalized for depression? What would you say if your friends asked where your parent or sibling was?

3. How would you feel about taking a drug when its long-term safety has not yet been studied?

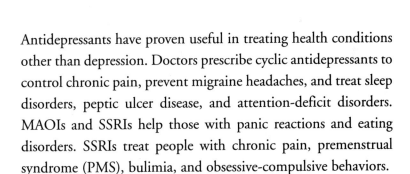

8

Other Uses for Antidepressants

Antidepressants have proven useful in treating health conditions other than depression. Doctors prescribe cyclic antidepressants to control chronic pain, prevent migraine headaches, and treat sleep disorders, peptic ulcer disease, and attention-deficit disorders. MAOIs and SSRIs help those with panic reactions and eating disorders. SSRIs treat people with chronic pain, premenstrual syndrome (PMS), bulimia, and obsessive-compulsive behaviors.

Fibromyalgia=Chronic Pain

Fibromyalgia is a common and painful arthritis-related condition that causes chronic muscle pain, fatigue, and poor sleep. Doctors have found that some tricyclic antidepressants restore deep sleep,

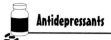

so that people wake up refreshed with increased energy and some pain relief. They should be taken in small doses, much less than those taken to treat depression.[1] SSRIs and SNRIs may also be helpful for those with fibromyalgia.

Premenstrual Syndrome (PMS)

For some women PMS is a monthly nightmare of tension, irritability, appetite changes, headaches, mood swings, and bloating. The current treatments for PMS, including diet, exercise, and hormones, often offer little or no relief. A 1995 Canadian study published in the *New England Journal of Medicine* reported that Prozac greatly reduced PMS symptoms with few side effects. Eli Lilly and Company, the manufacturer of Prozac, has not decided if it will go for Food and Drug Administration (FDA) approval for PMS. In the meantime, "a growing number of doctors have already been using Prozac to treat the worst cases of PMS."[2] Researchers do not know exactly how Prozac and other SSRIs antidepressants help PMS.

Kris (not her real name) was diagnosed with stress and depression resulting from or causing severe PMS. She began taking Zoloft, an SSRI antidepressant. She remembered:

> *It took Zoloft about four to six weeks to have a positive effect. I consider Zoloft a miracle drug in my condition. I don't have the temper edge anymore, things don't bother me as much, I can handle let downs a lot easier than I used to, and my PMS has eased considerably. This drug works!* [3]

Obsessive-Compulsive Disorder (OCD)

When Tom (not his real name) walks to school every morning, he has one rule—do not step on a sidewalk crack. If he does, he runs home and starts walking again. He is often late to school because of his obsessive-compulsive disorder (OCD).[4]

Tom and about 2.4 million other Americans have OCD. Typical obsessions include a fear of dirt and germs, fear of acting on violent or aggressive feelings, feeling overly concerned for others' safety, and over-concern with order and arrangement. Although these obsessions are disturbing, the person cannot shut them off. Compulsions are rituals that do not make sense, but that the person feels compelled to perform over and over. Typical compulsions include washing, cleaning, counting, arranging, checking, saving, and repeating. Compulsions are often linked to obsessions.[5]

When some experts thought this disorder was partially a brain chemistry problem, researchers turned to antidepressants for help. Their hunch paid off and the FDA now approves Prozac, Luvox, and Anafranil to treat OCD.

The antidepressant Prozac, said Delores (not her real name), has changed her life. Delores was compulsive about keeping her life in order. She often did laundry every night because she could not stand to see dirty clothes. She constantly checked the stove and coffeepot to make sure they were not on when she left for work. Because she could not tolerate any papers on her desk, she would work until 11 P.M., then come back three hours later to get a headstart on the next day. Friends were never invited to her house because they dirtied her glasses.[6]

The former secretary went through twenty-five years of psychotherapy but found that it did not help. Next Delores tried

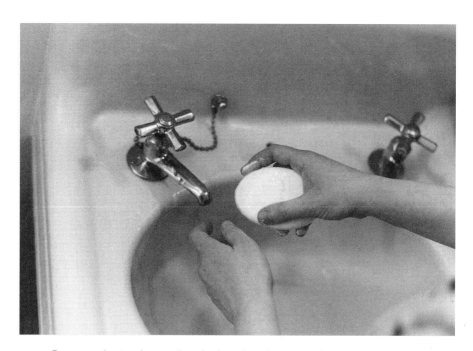

Because she is obsessed with the idea that everything she touches is covered with germs, this woman washes her hands many times a day. Taking an antidepressant will weaken her obsessive thoughts and the urge to compulsively wash her hands.

Nardil, an MAOI. But when she took this antidepressant with cheese and allergy pills, she had a heart attack. Her husband eventually walked out and she realized she had lost fourteen jobs. She started taking Prozac™ and her life finally changed. Her only side effect has been heavy sweating. "I'm nowhere near prefect," she said. "But it's a big, big improvement. Prozac has really been a godsend to me."[7]

Animal psychologists and veterinarians sometimes prescribe low doses of Prozac to treat dogs and cats with OCD. In the United States, over 1 million dogs are estimated to have this disorder.[8] One dog with OCD, for example, barked constantly at any light, whether it was sunlight streaming in a window or light reflecting off a shiny surface. Prozac helped the dog not react to light, and once again, the dog's owners are enjoying their pet and a quiet home.

Another pet owner brought her cat to the veterinarian. The cat was chewing patches of fur off her back and vomiting a lot. The vet explained that "the cat had grown depressed and self-absorbed."[9] The cat was put on feline-sized doses of Prozac.

Prozac, though, cannot cure a dog or cat of OCD. Explained Dr. Robert Schick from the University of Pennsylvania School of Veterinary Medicine, "As soon as a dog is taken off the medication, the problem comes right back."[10] But pet owners find that the drug helps. One dog owner, after trying many therapies for her golden retriever with OCD, said that after her dog began taking Prozac, she saw a definite change. Now, he's a very happy dog. And it makes me feel better too."[11]

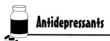

Panic Attacks and Phobias

For years, Alison (not her real name) was nearly a prisoner in her own house. She could not leave unless her husband came with her. But after taking Prozac for three months, the symptoms of her disorder (called agoraphobia) have disappeared. "I feel like I'm part of the world again," Alison said.[12] Alison and others who experience panic attacks, phobias, and agoraphobia can be helped with therapy and antidepressant medication.

Sleep Disorders

Doctors sometimes prescribe tricyclic antidepressants such as Elavil to improve sleep. These drugs work by allowing the sleeping brain to spend more time in the deep or restorative phase of sleep. During deep sleep, the brain restores neurotransmitters and the muscles fully relax. The tricyclic drugs are taken in low dosages, usually $\frac{1}{10}$ to $\frac{1}{20}$ the amount needed to treat depression. Because the medication produces drowsiness within thirty to sixty minutes, people often take their antidepressant just before bedtime.

Bulimia

Uncommon in men, bulimia nervosa is a chronic eating disorder. This disease affects nearly 3 percent of American women, usually between ages eighteen to thirty-five.[13] Symptoms include reccurring binge eating, feelings of lack of control, self-induced vomiting, use of laxatives or diuretics (water pills), strict dieting, fasting, rigorous exercise to prevent weight gain, and over-concern with body shape and weight. Two tricyclic antidepressants, Elavil and Tofranil, and the MAOIs have been used to treat people with bulimia. In April 1994 the FDA approved Prozac to treat bulimia.

Attention Deficit Hyperactivity Disorder (ADHD)

One of the most common behavioral disorders in American children, Attention Deficit Hyperactivity Disorder (ADHD) affects about 3.5 million American children.[14] One third to two thirds of ADHD children continue to have the same symptoms when they are adults.[15] People with ADHD are easily distracted, extremely impulsive, and hyperactive so that sitting still is nearly impossible.

In 1937, a Rhode Island doctor found that giving stimulants to ADHD children calmed them down. By the mid-1970s, one stimulant, Ritalin[TM], had become the most prescribed drug for ADHD. Sometimes a combination of a stimulant and an antidepressant is prescribed, but for others an antidepressant alone such as Prozac or Zoloft is effective. Three antidepressants—Tofranil, Norpamin, and Elavil—can help decrease hyperactivity and aggression in some young people with ADHD.

Bright Outlook for Antidepressants

Researchers continue to perform studies to see if antidepressants can treat other problems. For example, two recent studies found that Zoloft seems to help people suffering from severe shyness. Although these preliminary results are promising, more research is needed.

New antidepressants are being developed, too. The Pharmaceutical Research and Manufacturers of America has

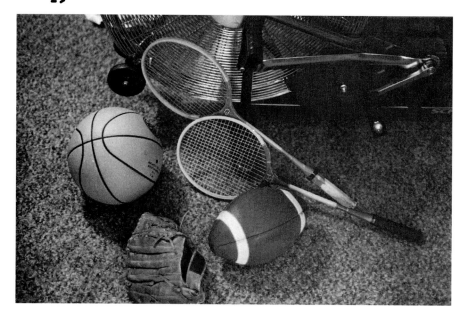

Exercise produces a sense of well-being and is an excellent supplement to antidepressant medication.

reported that thirteen new drugs for treating depression and other mood disorders, such as bipolar disorder, will soon go to the FDA for approval. With these future drugs and the many antidepressants now available, the future looks promising for those with depression and other disorders.

If you or someone you know is suffering from depression, the *Where to Go for Help* section at the end of this book provides names, addresses, and phone numbers of organizations that can provide help.

Questions for Discussion

1. Would you feel comfortable taking an antidepressant for a condition it was not originally created to treat? Why? Why not?

2. Exercise is an excellent supplement to antidepressant medication. Can you think of other ways to curb depression?

3. Can you think of any reasons why antidepressant side-effects vary from person to person?

Chapter Notes

Chapter 1

1. Edwin E. Aldrin, Jr., and Wayne Warga, *Return to Earth* (New York: Random House, 1973), p. 281.

2. Ibid., p. 300.

3. Marilynn Larkin, "Inevitable Companions? Depression & Advancing Age," *FDA Consumer,* March 1993, p. 18.

4. Ibid.

5. Personal interview with Kent, September 20, 1995.

6. Robert Campbell, *The Enigma of the Mind* (New York: Time-Life Books, 1976), p. 66.

7. U.S. Department of Health and Human Serivices, Public Health Service, National Institute of Mental Health, *Depressive Illnesses: Treatments Bring New Hope* (Rockville, Md.: 1994), p. 1.

8. Ibid.

9. Personal interview with Cathy, August 25, 1995.

10. Erica E. Goode, et al. "Beating Depression," *U.S. News & World Report*, March 5, 1990, pp. 50–51, 53.

11. "Facts and Figures on Depression," Great Neck, N.Y.: National Alliance for Research on Schizophrenia and Depression (NARSAD, 1995). Unpaged.

12. Ibid.

13. American Association of Suicidology, "Understanding and Preventing Suicide," pamphlet (Washington, D.C.: 1996).

14. "Facts and Figures on Depression," Great Neck, N.Y.: National Alliance for Research on Schizophrenia and Depression (NARSAD, 1995).

15. "Depression. A Flaw in Chemistry, not Character," poster, National Alliance for Research on Schizophrenia and Depression, Summer 1995.

16. "Facts and Figures on Depression," Great Neck, N.Y.: National Alliance for Research on Schizophrenia and Depression (NARSAD, 1995).

Chapter 2

1. Richard M. Restak, *The Mind* (New York: Bantam Books, 1988), pp. 182–183.

2. Ibid., p. 183.

3. Mark S. Gold, *Wonder Drugs: How They Work* (New York: Pocket Books, 1987), p. 109.

4. Jack Engler and Daniel Goleman, *The Consumer's Guide to Psychotherapy* (New York: Simon & Schuster, 1992), p. 619.

5. Mary H. Cooper, "Prozac Controversy" *CQ Researcher*, August 25, 1994, p. 731.

6. Ibid., p. 733.

7. Ibid.

8. Tracy Thompson, "The Wizard of Prozac," *Readers Digest*, October 1994, p. 73.

Chapter 3

1. Sandra Salmans, *Depression: Questions You Have . . . Answers You Need* (Allentown, Pa.: People's Medical Society, 1995), p. 119.

2. Colette Dowling, *You Mean I Don't Have to Feel This Way? New Help for Depression, Anxiety, and Addiction* (New York: Charles Scribners Sons, 1991), p. 189.

3. Debra Elfenbein, ed., *Living with Prozac and other Selective Serotonin Reuptake Inhibitors* (SSRIs): *Personal Accounts of Life on Antidepressants* (San Francisco: Harper, 1995), p. 57.

4. Ibid.

5. Dowling, p. 189.

6. Ibid.

7. Erica E. Goode, et al., "Tailoring Treatment for Depression's Many Forms," *U.S News & World Report*, March 5, 1990, p. 54.

8. Jack Engler and Daniel Goleman, *The Consumer's Guide to Psychotherapy* (New York: Simon & Schuster, 1992), p. 611.

9. Ibid.

10. Personal interview with Chuck, September 10, 1995.

11. Patricia L. Owen, *I Can See Tomorrow: A Guide for Living with Depression* (Center City, Minn.: Hazelden Foundation, 1995), p. 89.

12. Ibid., pp. 89, 90.

13. Ibid., p. 93.

14. Ibid., p. 110.

15. Salmans, pp.120–121.

16. Dowling, p. 193.

17. American Pharmaceutical Association, *Therapeutic Options in the Treatment of Depression: A Continuing Education Program for Pharmacists* (Washington, D.C., 1994), p. 6.

18. Salmans, p. 121.

19. American Psychiatric Association, *Depression* (Washington, D.C., March, 1, 1994), p. 8.

20. Marilyn Larkin, "Depression and Advancing Age," *FDA Consumer*, Washington, D.C.: March 1993, p. 20.

21. Anne Brown, "Current Developments in the Treatment of Depression—A Special Report," *NARSAD Research Newsletter*, Spring 1995, pp. 19–20.

22. Ibid., p. 20.

23. James W. Long and James J. Rybacki, *The Essential Guide to Prescription Drugs* (New York: Haper Perennial, 1994), p. 56.

24. Owen, pp. 99–100.

25. Mark S. Gold and Lois B. Morris, *The Good News about Depression: Cures and Treatments in the New Age of Psychiatry* (New York: Bantam Books, 1995), p. 294.

26. Ibid., pp. 292–293.

27. Ibid., p. 293.

28. Ibid.

29. "ABCs of Antidepressants," *USA Today,* (newsletter), February 1993, p. 12.

30. Salmans, p. 96.

31. Ibid.

32. Anne Brown, "Current Developments in the Treatment of Depression: A Special Report," *NARSAD Research Newsletter,* Spring 1995, p. 18.

33. Kathy Cronkite, *On the Edge of Darkness: Conversations about Conquering Depression* (New York: Doubleday, 1994), p. 186.

34. Salmans, p. 122.

35. American Pharmaceutical Association, "Therapeutic Options in the Treatment of Depression," (Washington, D.C.: APA, 1994), p. 11.

36. Salmans, p. 124.

37. Colette Dowling, *You Mean I Don't Have to Feel This Way?,* (New York: Charles Scribner's Sons, 1991,) p. 22.

38. Geoffrey Cowley et. al., "The Promise of Prozac," *Newsweek*, March 26, 1990, p. 39.

39. Sasha Nemecek, "Backfire," *Scientific American,* September, 1994, p. 23.

40. Brown, p. 20.

Chapter 4

1. The National Alliance for the Mentally Ill, "Depressive Disorders in Children and Adolescents," pamphlet (Arlington, Va.: NAMI Medical Information Series, 1992), p.1.

2. Lawrence L. Kerns and Adrienne Lieberman, *Helping Your Depressed Child* (Rocklin, Calif.: Prima Publishing, 1993), p. xiii.

3. Colette Dowling, *You Mean I Don't Have to Feel This Way?* (New York: Charles Scribners Sons, 1991), p. 128.

4. Personal interview with Dr. Ralph Rovner, clinical psychologist, Edina, Minn., June 26, 1995.

5. Beth Brophy, "Kindergarten in the Prozac Nation: Are There Risks in Giving Kids Antidepressants?," *U.S. News & World Report,* New York: November 13, 1995, p. 96–97.

6. Ibid.

7. Ibid.

8. Ibid., p. 97

9. Ibid.

10. Dowling, p. 129.

11. Ibid.

12. Ibid., pp. 129–130.

13. Kerns and Lieberman, pp. 210–211.

14. Ibid., p. 211.

15. Ibid., pp. 211–212.

16. Sandra Arbetter, "Depression: Way Beyond the Blues," *Current Health 2*, December 1993, pp. 5–6.

17. The Associated Press, "Suicide Rates Up Among Some," (New York: Wireready Newswire Systems, Inc., April 21, 1995).

18. American Academy of Child & Adolescent Psychiatry, "Teen Suicide," fact sheet, (Washington, D.C.: Facts for Families Problem Series, October 1992).

19. Anne Brown, "Mood Disorders in Children and Adolescents," *NARSAD Research Newsletter,* Winter 1996, p. 13.

20. Kerns, p. 129.

21. The Associated Press, "Suicide Rates Up Among Some," (New York: Wireready Newswire Systems, Inc., April 24, 1995), p. 43.

22. Arbetter, p. 7.

23. Ibid.

24. Ibid.

25. Ibid.

Chapter 5

1. American Pharmaceutical Association, "APhA Special Report: Therapeutic Options in the Treatment of Depression," (Washington, D.C., 1994). Unpaged.

2. American Pharmaceutical Association, *Therapeutic Options in the Treatment of Depression,* Washington: APA, 1994, pp. 9–10.

3. Jack Engler and Daniel Goleman, *The Consumer's Guide to Psychotherapy* (New York: Simon & Schuster, 1992), p. 611.

4. Lawrence L. Kerns and Adrienne B. Lieberman, *Helping Your Depressed Child* (Rocklin, Calif.: Prima Publishing, 1993), p. 212.

5. American Pharmaceutical Association, *Therapeutic Options in the Treatment of Depression* (Washington, D.C.: APA, 1994), p. 9.

6. Ibid., p. 10.

7. Sandra Salmans, *Depression: Questions You Have . . . Answers You Need* (Allentown, Pa.: People's Medical Society, 1995), p. 127.

8. Ibid.

9. Anne Brown, "Current Developments in the Treatment of Depression—A Special Report," *NARSAD Research Newsletter,* Spring 1995, pp. 19–20.

10. A. John Rush, et. al., *Depression in Primary Care: Volume 2, Treatment of Major Depression* (Rockville, Md: Agency for Health Care Policy and Research, 1993), p. 1111.

Chapter 6

1. Donald L. Klein and Paul H. Wender, *Understanding Depression: A Complete Guide to Its Diagnosis and Treatment* (New York: Oxford University Press, 1993), p. 133.

2. Mark S. Gold, *The Good News about Depression* (New York: Bantam Books, 1995), p. 274.

3. Philip Elmer-DeWitt, "Depression: The Growing Role of Drug Therapies," *Time,* July 6, 1992, p. 57.

4. Ibid.

5. Jack Engler and Daniel Coleman, *The Consumer's Guide to Psychotherapy* (New York: Simon & Schuster, 1993), p. 617.

6. Klein and Wender, pp. 159–161.

7. Ibid., p. 160.

8. Gold, p. 275.

9. Jack M. Gorman, *The Essential Guide to Psychiatric Drugs* (New York: St. Martin's Press, 1990), p. 83.

10. American Pharmaceutical Association, *Therapeutic Options in the Treatment of Depression* (Washington, D.C.: APA, 1994), pp. 6, 9.

11. Klein and Wender, p. 134.

Chapter 7

1. Sandra Arbetter, "Depression: Way Beyond the Blues," *Current Health 2,* December 1993, p. 5.

2. Peter D. Kramer, "The Transformation of Personality," *Psychology Today,* July/August 1993, pp. 45–46.

3. Sandra Salmans, *Depression: Questions You Have . . . Answers You Need* (Allentown, Pa.: People's Medical Society, 1995), p. 135.

4. Ronald R. Fieve, *Prozac: Questions and Answers for Patients, Family, and Physicians* (New York: Avon Books, 1994), pp. 131–132.

5. Salmans, p. 135.

6. Ibid., p. 132.

7. Fieve, pp. 92–93.

8. Demitri Papolos and Janice Papolos, *Overcoming Depression* (New York: Harper Perrenials, 1992), pp. 160–161.

9. Lawrence Mondi, "Did Prozac Make Him Do It?" *Time,* November 28, 1994, p. 66.

10. James J. Rybacki and James W. Long, *The Essential Guide to Prescription Drugs* (New York: HarperCollins Publishers, 1996), p. 409.

11. Jack Engler and Daniel Goleman, *The Consumer's Guide to Psychotherapy* (New York: Simon & Schuster, 1992), p. 611.

12. Debra Elfenbein, *Living with Prozac and Other Selective Serotonin-Reuptake Inhibitors* (San Francisco: HarperCollins Publisher, 1995), p. 193.

13. Ibid., p. 20.

14. Ibid., pp. 20–22.

15. Ibid., p. 244.

16. Ibid., pp. 248–249.

17. American Pharmaceutical Association, *APhA Special Report: Therapeutic Options in the Treatment of Depression,* booklet (Washington, D.C., 1994), p. 12.

18. Elfenbein, pp. 155–156.

19. A. John Rush, et. al., *Depression in Primary Care: Vol. II, Treatment of Major Depression* (Rockville, Md.: Agency for Health Care Policy and Research, Public Health Service, U.S. Department of Health and Human Services, April 1993), p. 3.

20. Ibid.

Chapter 8

1. Mary Anne Dunkin and Marcy O'Koon, "The Drug Guide," *Arthritis Today,* July/August 1995, p. 38.

2. "A New Use for Prozac," *Newsweek,* June 19, 1995, p. 85.

3. Personal interview with Kris, August 21, 1995.

4. Robert Taibbi, "More Than Just Nerves: Understanding Obsessive-Compulsive Disorders & Panic Attacks," *Current Health 2,* December 1994, p. 13.

5. Mary H. Cooper, "Prozac and the Treatment of Serious Mental Illness" *CQ Researcher,* August 19, 1994, p. 726.

6. Geoffrey Cowley et al., "The Promise of Prozac," *Newsweek,* March 26, 1990, p. 41.

7. Ibid.

8. *20/20* Weekly television show, aired 9:00 P.M. Central Time, Friday, March 22, 1996.

9. Elizabeth Wurtzel, *Prozac Nation: Young and Depressed in America* (Boston: Houghton Mifflin Company, 1994), p. 295.

10. "Prozac Ration: Is This the Answer for Compulsive Canines?" *People's Weekly,* October 17, 1994, p. 92.

11. Ibid.

12. Jeffrey M. Jones and Ron Schaumburg, *Everything You Need to Know About Prozac* (New York: Bantam Books, 1991), p. 88.

13. LynNell Hancock, "Mother's Little Helper," *Newsweek,* March 18, 1996, p. 52.

14. Claudia Wallis, "Life in Overdrive," *Time,* July 18, 1994, p. 43.

15. Ibid., p. 44.

Where to Go for Help

Many organizations offer information about depression, including treatment and support.

Information: Depression

American Academy of Child and Adolescent Psychiatry
3615 Wisconsin Avenue, NW
Washington, DC 20016-3007
(202) 966-7300
Provides information.

American Association for Marriage and Family Therapy
1133 15th Street NW
Suite 300
Washington, DC 20005
(800) 374-2638
Provides referrals.

American Psychiatric Association
1400 K Street, NW
Washington, DC 20005
(202) 682-6220
Provides information and referrals.

American Psychological Association
750 First Street NE
Washington, DC 20002
(800) 374-3120
Provides information and referrals.

Depression After Delivery (DAD)
P.O. Box 1282
Morrisville, PA 19067
(215) 295-3994
Provides information.

National Alliance for the Mentally Ill (NAMI)
200 N. Glebe Road, Suite 1015
Arlington, VA 22203-3754
(800) 950-6264
Provides information and referrals.

National Alliance for Research on Schizophrenia and Depression (NARSAD)
60 Cutter Mill Road, Suite 200
Great Neck, NY 11021
(516) 829-0091
Provides information and referrals.

National Association of Social Workers
750 First Street NE
Suite 700
Washington, DC 20002
(202) 408-8600
Provides referrals.

National Depressive and Manic Depressive Association
730 North Franklin
Suite 501
Chicago, IL 60620
(800) 826-3632
Provides information and referrals.

National Institutes of Mental Health
Room 10-85
5600 Fishers Lane
Rockville, MD 20857
(800) 421-4211
Provides information.

National Mental Health Association (NMHA)
1201 Prince Street
Alexandria, VA 22314-2971
(800) 969-6642
Provides information and referrals.

Treatment and Support: Depression

Emotional Health Anonymous
P.O. Box 63236
Los Angeles, CA 90063-0236
(213) 268-7220
Self-help programs.

Emotions Anonymous
P.O. Box 4245
St. Paul, MN 55104-0245
(612) 647-9712
Self-help programs.

National Foundation for Depressive Illness
P.O. Box 2257
New York, NY 10116
(800) 248-4344

Information: Suicide

Suicide Awareness Voices of Education (SAVE)
P.O. Box 24507
Minneapolis, MN 55424
(612) 946-7998
e-mail address:
save@winternet.com
Provides information.

Glossary

addict—Someone who is dependent on or controlled by a drug.

agoraphobia—The fear of large, open spaces.

antidepressant medication—A medication prescribed to treat depression.

antihistamines—Medications that relieve the symptoms of allergies or colds by blocking the production or action of histamines.

anxiety—A feeling of unease and distress that may not be related to any particular object or situation.

behavioral therapy—This therapy helps people change and gain control over their unwanted behaviors.

bipolar disorder—A mental illness that causes extreme mood swings from intense excitement and happiness to deep sadness.

bulimia—An eating disorder in which a person periodically gorges on food and induces vomiting.

cyclic antidepressant—A class of antidepressants used to treat depression and other disorders.

depression—A period in which a person feels hopeless, sad, and in despair.

dosage—Amount of an antidepressant medication prescribed by a doctor.

episode of depression—The period of time during which a person is depressed.

fibromyalgia—Painful arthritis-related condition. People with fibromyalgia have chronic muscle pain, fatigue, and poor sleep.

generic drugs—Similar to the brand-name drug, but with small differences.

genetics—A branch of biology dealing with heredity.

hallucination—Imaginary sights, sounds, and smells believed to be real.

histamines—Substances released by the body that cause runny, itchy eyes and a runny nose during allergy attacks or colds.

mania—A period of abnormally intense excitement, hyperactivity, rapid shifting of ideas, and lack of sleep.

manic-depressive—See bipolar disorder.

monoamine oxidase inhibitors (MAOIs)—a class of antidepressants used to treat depression and other disorders.

mood brighteners—Antidepressants that seem to enhance healthy, normal people's lives.

neurotransmitter—A chemical substance that relays messages between nerves.

norepinephrine—A brain chemical that affects mood and behavior.

obsessive compulsive disorder (OCD)—A condition in which someone has a distressing set of repetitive thoughts and/or actions.

overdose—An excessive or lethal dose of a drug.

panic attack—Sudden, unexplained occasions when someone feels overwhelming fear, though there is nothing to cause fear.

phobia—An irrational, intense fear of an object or situation.

premenstrual syndrome (PMS)—Prior to menstruation, some women experience irritablity, anxiety, tiredness, headaches, and bloating.

prescription—A doctor's orders or instructions for a drug.

psychiatrist—A physician specializing in mental illness. He or she is licensed to prescribe medications.

psychiatry—The medical study, diagnosis, treatment, and prevention of mental illness.

relapse—The reoccurrence of a disease after a period of recovery.

Ritalin—A stimulant medication used to treat attention deficit hyperactivity disorder.

schizophrenia—A group of severe mental disorders in which a person loses awareness of reality and the ability to relate closely with others. The person often shows behavior problems and lacks the ability to reason well.

selective serotonin reuptake inhibitors (SSRIs)—A class of antidepressants used to treat depression and other disorders.

serotonin—A brain chemical that affects mood and behavior.

serotonin nonselective reuptake inhibitors (SNRIs)—A class of antidepressants used to treat depression and other disorders.

side effects—The unintended, but fairly common effects from taking a medication.

suicide—Voluntary, intentional taking of one's life.

synapse—The gap between nerves.

therapy—Treatment to help someone get over an illness, disability, or other conditions such as phobias.

tyramine—A substance found in some food and beverages that tends to increase the heart rate.

washout period—Period of time to allow the body to washout or remove any traces of an antidepressant.

withdrawal—The process of ridding the body of a drug.

Further Reading

Depression

Carter, Sharon. *Coping with Depression.* New York: The Rosen Publishing Group, 1990.

Cronkite, Kathy. *On the Edge of Darkness: Conversations About Conquering Depression.* New York: Doubleday, 1994.

Cush, Cathie. *Depression.* New York: Steck-Vaughn Company, 1994.

Dowling, Collette. *You Mean I Don't Have to Feel This Way?* New York: Charles Scribner's Sons, 1991.

Duke, Patty, and Gloria Hochman. *A Brilliant Madness: Living with Manic-Depressive Illness.* New York: Bantam Books, 1992.

Elfenbein, Debra. *Living with Prozac and Other Selective Serotonin Reuptake Inhibitors (SSRIs).* San Francisco: Harper, 1995.

Gold, Mark, and Lois B. Morris. *The Good News About Depression: Cures and Treatments in the New Age.* New York: Bantam Books, 1995.

Greist, John H., and James W. Jefferson. *Depression and Its Treatment.* New York: Warner Books, 1992.

Kerns, Lawrence L., and Adrienne B. Lieberman. *Helping Your Depressed Child.* Rocklin, Calif.: Prima Publishing, 1993.

Klein, Donald F., and Paul H. Wender. *Understanding Depression: A Complete Guide to Its Diagnosis and Treatment.* New York: Oxford University Press, 1993.

Knauth, Percy. *A Season in Hell.* New York: Harper & Row, 1975.

Maloney, Michael, and Rachel Kranz. *Straight Talk about Anxiety and Depression.* New York: Facts on File, 1991.

Owens, Patricia L. *I Can See Tomorrow: A Guide for Living with Depression.* Center City, Minn: Hazelden Foundation, 1995.

Papolos, Demitri, and Janice Papolos. *Overcoming Depression.* New York: HarperPerennial, 1992.

Robbins, Paul R. *Understanding Depression.* Jefferson, N.C.: McFarland & Company, 1993.

Salmans, Sandra. *Depression: Questions You Have . . . Answers You Need.* Allentown, Pa.: People's Medical Society, 1995.

Silverstein, Herma. *Teenage Depression.* New York: Franklin Watts, 1990.

Wurtzel, Elizabeth. *Prozac Nation: Young and Depressed in America.* Boston: Houghton Mifflin Company, 1994.

Drugs Used to Treat Depression

Fieve, Ronald R. *Prozac.* New York: Avon Books, 1994.

Jonas, Jeffrey M., and Ron Schaumburg. *Everything You Need to Know about Prozac.* New York: Bantam Books, 1991.

Long, James W., and James J. Rybacki. *The Essential Guide to Prescription Drugs.* New York: HarperCollins, 1995.

Salzman, Bernard. *The Handbook of Psychiatric Drugs.* New York: Henry Holt and Company, 1991.

Yudofsky, Stuart, and Tom Ferguson. *What You Need to Know about Psychiatric Drugs.* Washington, D.C.: American Psychiatric Press, 1991.

Suicide

Ayan, Eleanor. *Teen Suicide: Is It Too Painful to Grow Up?* New York: Twenty First Century Books, 1993.

Crook, Marian. *Please Listen to Me!* Bellingham, Wash.: Self-Counsel Press, 1992.

Galas, Judith. *Teen Suicide.* San Diego: Lucent Books, 1994.

Lester, David. *The Enigma of Adolescent Suicide.* Philadelphia: The Charles Press, 1993.

Smith, Judie. *Coping with Suicide.* New York: Rosen Publishing Group, 1990.

Index

Eli Lilly and Company, 21, 22, 89, 100
Emslie, Dr. Graham, 53

F
fibromyalgia, 99–100
fluoxetine, *See* Prozac™
Food and Drug Administration (FDA), 13, 21, 22–23, 45, 51, 89, 94, 100, 101, 105, 106
Freedman, Dr. Daniel X., 27
Fuller, Ray, 21

G
Gelwan, Elliot, 69
Gold, Dr. Mark S., 37, 74–75, 78
Gold, Dr. Philip, 87

H
Hazelden Foundation, 30
Hemingway, Earnest, 18
Hippocrates, 17
histamines, 22
Holland, Dr. Jimmie, 44

I
imipramine, *See* Tofranil™

J
jaundice, 21

K
Kerns, Dr. Lawrence L., 48, 65
Klein, Dr. Donald L., 74, 83
Kline, Dr. Nathan, 20
Kuhn, Dr. Roland, 19

L
Luvox™, 101

M
mania, 54–55
MAOIs
  chemical action, 42
  combinations, 40

history, 20–21
interactions, 81, 82, 94
selection, 75–76, 60
side effects, 74, 76, 78–81
treatment, 33, 40, 81–82, 85, 104–105
migraine headaches, 99
Molloy, Bryan B., 21
Musicante, Ruth, 54

N
National Alliance for the Mentally Ill (NAMI), 48,53
National Alliance for Research on Schizophrenia and Depression (NARSAD), 12,46
National Institute of Mental Health (NIMH), 12, 36, 46, 87, 88
nefazodone, *See* Serzone™
neurotransmitters, 42
norepinephrine, 42
Norpamin™, 105
nortriptyline, *See* Pamelor™

O
obsessive-compulsive disorder (OCD), 49, 53, 99, 101, 103
Owen, Dr. Patricia, 30

P
Pamelor™, 63
panic attacks, 33, 99, 104
paroxetine, *See* Paxil™
Paxil™, 23, 36, 53, 85, 92–93, 97
Pfizer, Inc., 23
Pharmaceutical Research and Manufacturers of America, 105–106
phobias, 33
Plath, Sylvia, 18
post-achievement depression, 6
premenstrual syndrome (PMS), 99, 100–101
Prozac™, 22–23, 39, 41, 44, 53, 61, 85, 86–87, 89, 92, 97, 10, 101, 103, 105